Tender Loving Greed
2009 Notes

Tender Loving Greed
2009 Notes

By Mary Adelaide Mendelson
&
Walton Mendelson

One-Off Press
Prescott, Arizona
2009

To:
Mary Adelaide Mendelson
Petey Cerf
Mary Bush

Table of Contents

PART ONE

Tender Loving Greed—1974

TENDER LOVING GREED

MARY ADELAIDE MENDELSON

How the
Incredibly Lucrative
NURSING HOME
"INDUSTRY" Is
Exploiting America's
Old People and
Defrauding Us All

Why, with an annual $3.5 billion pouring into nursing homes, is there practically no such thing as an excellent nursing home in America today?

Why did nursing home stocks provide a spectacular stock-promoters' bonanza comparable to the Florida Land Boom?

Why, with one million Americans currently in nursing homes, and with the appalling conditions documented again and again in congressional hearings and in the media, does nothing seem to change?

In this book the answers are at last provided. After ten years of intensive investigation, Mary Adelaide Mendelson here exposes the inner workings of the "industry" that talks Tender Loving Care and Happiness Benefits while it mistreats the old and the helpless and, swallowing our tax money, robs us all. Cutting through a jungle of financial and legal, business and government operations, she uncovers the core of a national scandal: how the very munificence of government aid, together with the lack of effective government control, has made the nursing home industry into a giant profit machine which has attracted not only thousands of small-time hustlers but, much more importantly and ominously, the big-money manipulators.

Among the revelations:

- How numerous nursing homes get away with stealing patients' social security checks and their pin money and extorting extra money from worried relatives.
- The two prominent Massachusetts attorneys general who failed to act on the evidence of improper financial dealings placed before them . . . The governor of Ohio who failed to obtain the extradition of the criminally indicted nursing home owner who is now operating freely in Louisiana.
- Political contributions from nursing home interests ... The administrators who shuttle between jobs in

Tender Loving Greed

Tender Loving Greed

How the Incredibly Lucrative
Nursing Home "Industry" Is Exploiting
America's Old People and
Defrauding Us All

By Mary Adelaide Mendelson

ALFRED A. KNOPF / New York
1974

THIS IS A BORZOI BOOK
PUBLISHED BY ALFRED A. KNOPF, INC.

Copyright © 1974 by Mary Adelaide Mendelson

Library of Congress Cataloging in Publication Data

Mendelson, Mary Adelaide.
Tender loving greed.
i. Nursing homes—United States.   I. Title.
[DNLM: i. Nursing homes—U.S.—Popular works.
WT27 AAi M4f   1974]
RA998.U6M46   1974   362.6'11'60973   73-17312
ISBN 0-394-47597-6

Manufactured in the United States of America

FIRST EDITION

To those dedicated civil servants
who are an exception to what is said
in the pages that follow

CONTENTS

ACKNOWLEDGMENTS

The acknowledgments for this book could easily become impossibly long, since over the years of its preparation I have depended upon many persons in many different ways. To most of those who have assisted, my very sincere, even if wordless, thanks. But there are some whose contributions simply cannot be passed over in silence. First among these is David Hapgood, whose help was immeasurable. It was he who made sense out of the massive collection of my material, selecting what was truly pertinent and culling the essential points from my often rambling tales.

In my travels around the country, I met an occasional civil servant who truthfully answered my questions and, most important, a few who furnished key documents that are the substantiating material for some of the charges in the book. Most of these persons have chosen to remain anonymous, lest public disclosure of their assistance to me jeopardize their jobs. Two names only must serve to represent the many nameless civil servants to whom I am indebted: Frank C. Frantz, a deputy commissioner at the Department of Health, Education, and Welfare, and Sarah Skurrow, director of welfare audits in the Ohio Department of State Auditor.

Advice on finding my way through the legal and financial mazes of the nursing home industry has been constantly available from William D. Ginn Esq., of Thompson, Hine and Flory, and James F. McKenna, CPA, of Whitney Hill & Co. Friends have assisted me in collecting material, answering technical questions, visiting nursing homes, writing, criticizing, and typing copy. A few of these friends are Peggy Gokay,

· ACKNOWLEDGMENTS

Joanne Kaufman, Jane King, Patricia Kelley, Phyllis Jones, and Sally Lampee.

From my mother's estate, I received the financial freedom essential for traveling throughout the country. My mother herself became a nursing home patient several years after I started my work in the field, and her experience as a private paying patient in a philanthropic home left an indelible mark on this book. Although her story is never mentioned in what follows, the experiences of other patients and some nursing home employees do appear. In all such instances, the names have been changed, since identification could serve no purpose and might do harm. All other names used are factual.

Finally, very special thanks go to my husband Ralph, who has suffered with and for me over these ten years. His patience has been matched by his constancy in assistance. I can only wonder what the most liberated man or woman might do without an endless supply of tolerance from a spouse.

M. A. M.

PREFACE

This book is an indictment of the conditions widely prevalent in the American nursing home industry as well as an examination of the reasons those conditions prevail. It is also an indictment of those who profit unreasonably from these conditions. Finally, it is an indictment of government—federal, state and local—for its failure to regulate the industry. It is based on ten years of intensive research, of visits to homes of every size and type, of countless interviews with nursing home operators, with government regulators, with patients and relatives.

Those connected with the industry and those charged with its regulation will see it as an extremely severe indictment, and it comes as no surprise that already—in advance of publication—counterattacks are being mounted.

Nursing home operators will say that the evidence cited of poor care and high profits applies only to "isolated instances." Of course, I have not—no one person has—seen all or even most of the 23,000 homes that make up the industry. Yet, on the basis of my visits to more than 200 homes in various parts of the country, of testimony I have heard given to congressional committees, and of my interviews with government regulators in many states, I have come across scant evidence or even hearsay of truly excellent facilities. Keeping in mind that "good" and "bad" are value judgments, and an institution that is proper for one kind of patient may be wrong for another, I am sure there must be some good, even excellent, homes somewhere. I am sure that I will hear about them, after this book is published, from the few fortunate readers who have found them. But this can bring little comfort to the hundreds of thousands of elderly people and their families who must choose between the dreadful and, at best, the mediocre.

Apologists for the industry will deny my charge that greed is the principal cause of poor patient care—that the increasing amount of public money, most of it from Medicaid, going into nursing homes is being used to produce higher profits rather than better living conditions for their inhabitants. It is true that not every nursing home makes unconscionable profits. Some homes *do* provide services far in excess of the legal requirements; some of the smaller, older homes are going out of business for financial reasons. But the fact remains that while adequate financial data concerning the costs and profitability of the industry as a whole does not exist, there is ample evidence, on the basis of public studies, of the extremely high profitability of many nursing homes and chains, and I have found over and over again that nursing home owners go to great lengths to hide their profits—legal and illegal—from public view.

Well-intentioned government officials and legislators will quite understandably resent the pessimistic view I take of their efforts, for no one likes to hear it said that his work is futile. Again and again, regulators have assured me that once they were armed with new legislation they would be able to move swiftly and effectively against nursing home abuses. In the past ten years, new laws *have* been passed, new regulations *have* been written. Yet, fundamentally, nothing has changed. Legislators will cite the recent enactment of H.R. 1 and its accompanying regulations as a dramatic breakthrough. Perhaps. But while H.R. 1 makes illegal some common abuses, many of those abuses have long been illegal (to little avail) under various state laws—and it is only too likely that so long as enforcement continues to lag far behind legislation, the new laws, like the old, will merely create the illusion of progress without its substance.

What of the new nursing homes? The buildings are prettier, the brochures are flashier, the language is more "professional." But conditions inside are not significantly different. If, in isolated cases, truly humane and effective facilities now exist, their proprietors will exempt themselves from my indictment while recognizing its overall validity.

Finally, I welcome the controversy that this book will arouse, if it results in a greater public awareness of the truth about the nursing homes in which one million of our people live. For the most important deprivation those people have suffered is the lack of active public concern.

Tender Loving Greed

1

The Shame of Nursing Homes: The Fraud of Tender Loving Care

IN SEPTEMBER OF 1964 I took the job that led to the writing of this book.

The Federation for Community Planning of Cleveland had received a grant to hire a part-time consultant on nursing homes for three years. The members of the federation, a voluntary group of social agencies, were upset over recurrent reports of the horrors taking place in the nursing homes of our area. They hired me to find ways to prevent those horrors, ways that, in their minds—as in the minds of most other people—would have to mean better state regulations and higher state payments for nursing home patients. And so I went to work.

My three-year undertaking has now lasted almost 10 years, my part-time job very quickly became full time, and the area I was assigned to survey—Cleveland and the state of Ohio—became merely a part of a nationwide study. My original goal, to improve nursing home care in Cleveland, has expanded into something radically different: a determination to document and expose a national scandal in which greedy nursing home operators are getting rich by exploiting helpless patients and extracting huge sums from governments—state and federal—that do not seem to care either about the patients or the taxpayers.

None of that was clear to me when I started. I knew next to nothing about nursing homes then. I was hired for the study because of my background in government; I had taught government in college and high school, and after years of involvement in civic affairs I knew my way around the bureaucracies and politicians of Cleveland. So, once hired, I set out to educate myself. Given a title, a desk, a telephone, and an office, I immediately left them all behind and went out to talk to everyone I could find who was connected with nursing homes.

My education began with the first meetings held by a committee of the federation that was to determine the goals of my job. At those first meetings I was presented with the evidence, though I did not fully understand it until later, of how well-intentioned citizens had completely swallowed the claims of the nursing home industry. The position of the owners has always been that nursing homes are poverty stricken; that if there is poor care it is because they do not get enough money from government for publicly supported patients; and that more money will produce the better patient care that everyone including the owners would like to see. That committee proceeded, without questioning those assumptions, to decide that our goal was to seek to increase state payments by $80 a month per patient and to work for more "realistic" regulation. The group acted on the basis of cost figures supplied by the nursing home owners themselves; no one asked what if anything would be bought with the extra $80; no one defined the meaning of "realistic" regulation.

The performance was typical of all too many citizen efforts to reform the nursing homes. A glance at the makeup of the committee is instructive. As citizen groups so often do, the federation had turned to the "experts," and as a result the committee was dominated by representatives of the industry. The members of the committee were almost all either nursing home operators, other health professionals (the chairman was from Blue Cross), or officials responsible for regulating nursing homes. It should have been obvious, but was not, that the operators would promote their own economic interests, that others in the health-care industry would support their colleagues, and that the officials would side more often than not with those they were supposed to regulate. The sad fact is that, even today, those realities are not borne in mind by citizen groups who want, as we did, to heal our sick nursing homes.

We reformers set out with our feet firmly planted on the wrong path, a path laid out for us by the industry itself. Had 1 stayed on that path, had I continued to accept the well-intentioned assumptions of those who hired me, there would have been no reason to write this book. Fortunately, my first experiences in the real world of the nursing home shattered the assumptions on which my work had begun. And no one did more to instruct me than the first nursing home operator I met, Sanford Novak.

Sandy Novak was a stocky, fast-talking man who had clawed his way up from nowhere in the nursing home business. He was, I learned later, typical of many operators who had started on a shoestring and become prosperous in the industry. Five years earlier, Novak had been running a small grocery in the Cleveland ghetto with his father and brother, and had delivered groceries to a woman who owned three nursing homes in the neighborhood. With a stake of $10,000 and a mortgage from the woman, who retired to Florida, Novak then bought her three homes with a total of 70 beds. By the time I met him, in 1964, he owned four homes with 244 beds and was, by the standards of that time, a big operator. He was known, to those whose origins were more genteel, as one of the "bad guys" in the industry.

I met Novak under a can of asparagus. The can, a very expensive grade-A brand, stood on the mantelpiece in his basement-dining room office as evidence of the fine food served in that nursing home. I was to see an equivalent symbol in many other homes. As for that home, when Novak bragged to me about the ways he saved money on food, I began to doubt that the can of asparagus would ever find its way to the kitchen. In another of his homes, Novak showed me the curtains that surrounded each bed to give patients a privacy enjoyed in few nursing homes. He stressed that these curtains really worked—"not like the usual curtains they put up to get past the inspector. One yank and they fall down." That, too, was a scene I saw many times: equipment of many kinds, installed to satisfy legal requirements, that either did not function or was never used.

As Sandy Novak drove me around to his nursing homes in his Cadillac (standard equipment in the business), his rapid-fire anecdotes and his remarkably frank opinions were opening my eyes to nursing home reality. He scoffed at the notion that other operators were losing money in the business. He himself was making plenty of money, he boasted, even though almost all his patients were on welfare. If the government raised its rates, he told me, the money would stay in the operators' pockets. It would not go to better patient care, nor to raising the wages operators pay their help, whose low pay is a major factor in the mistreatment of patients. He told me how nursing homes collect kickbacks from the pharmacies and funeral homes that get their business. An investigation of who owns nursing homes, he suggested, would turn up the fact that many supposed owners were merely fronts; there was "a lot of Las Vegas money" in the business, he said—but none of it in his operations.

Everything that Sandy Novak told me (about operators other than himself) was confirmed many times over in later years. In retrospect I realized why he was considered one of the "bad guys" in the business. Yet Novak was no greedier, and the homes he ran no worse, than those who considered themselves the "good guys"; in some ways Novak's homes were above average. Sandy's sin was that he was less hypocritical about what he was doing.

My next illuminating encounter, this time on the official side, was with the director of Aid for the Aged for Cuyahoga County. George Cameron was then close to his retirement, a man who had lived with frequent frustration in his work. Innumerable complaints about the mistreatment of nursing home patients had come across his desk, and he now realized that nothing he could do would stop that mistreatment from being repeated. Innocently, I suggested to him that more explicit and demanding government regulations would end that mistreatment. Mr. Cameron did not agree—and I now know that those undertaking a study of nursing homes often begin with that illusion. Legislators, congressmen, and even presidential advisers have voiced such a faith in the inherent powers of stiffened laws. More regulations are meaningless, Cameron told me, as long as existing regulations are not enforced.

Mr. Cameron said that regulations have little effect, sometimes serving only to anesthetize the public with a false assurance that government is doing its job. He catalogued the sins of nursing home owners, ranging from neglect of patients to fraudulent use of tax dollars. He produced complaining letters from patients and their families and outraged reports from welfare workers, then wearily recounted how those letters and complaints, passed on by him to state authorities, were routinely ignored. He brought out records listing the large monthly payments by state and federal governments to nursing homes, physicians, pharmacists, ambulance companies, and so on. In what Mr. Cameron said, in the records I reviewed, and in the county welfare files to which he gave me access, I learned these first lessons of my assignment: how little the quality of nursing home care is determined by the charges for that care, how government regulators ignore complaints reaching them, and how providers of goods and services often charge for nondelivered products and care.

I began to see the evidence of collusion among nursing home operators, doctors, caseworkers, and others in schemes to procure maximum reimbursement for patients needing only minimum care. Such collusion can—and does—make patients of some who do not belong in nursing homes at all. The chief regional counsel for the Veterans Administration told me he suspected that a feeder system existed between the Cuyahoga County Workhouse and nursing homes, with prisoners sometimes being classified by workhouse personnel as needing nursing home care as they finished serving their sentences. His suggestions were later echoed by a nursing home administrator who described the system whereby welfare patients—particularly those without families—were placed in nursing homes even if they were able to live independently.

Given free access to the files on 2,000 Aid for the Aged recipients, I studied 200 cases in depth, hoping to obtain a profile of the average nursing home patient. And while I did learn something about the patients, I learned even more about the system. Within those files lay clear evidence of those evils which I have since learned are to be found all over the United States.

Then I began to visit as many nursing homes as I could. Eventually two friends joined me in these visits, and as witnesses to each other we were able to check our recollections and impressions.

We made our share of mistakes. At one time we tried using a tape recorder concealed in a knitting bag, an action we justified on the grounds that no one was speaking to us in confidence. We had not been trained in the techniques of spying, however, and many a statement of nursing home conditions was drowned out by the tape's all-too-faithful recording of the sound of our footsteps or other background noises. We gave up the tape on the day that one of us bumped a nursing home administrator in the abdomen with the knitting bag. The recorder gave out a telltale beep, drawing from the administrator a suspicious look and the remark that we should watch our bags because the patients could not be trusted. I also experimented with a miniature camera. I snapped many pictures, but the only one that came out well was a portrait of a bedpan. Our technological failures mattered little, however, compared to our growing expertise in telling truth from fiction in a nursing home.

We learned how to check by observation what we were told by the staff. Most of the advice in how-to-pick-a-nursing-home manuals and articles consists of questions to be asked of the administrator of the home. But since most of what many administrators told us just was not true, we had to learn to plan our visits so we could check the administrators' claims against the evidence of our own eyes.

The quality of care depends more than anything else on the size, ability, and motivation of the staff. We first attempted to find out how many registered nurses, licensed practical nurses, and aides served on each shift, whether there was a doctor on call, and whether patients had access to the services of a dentist and podiatrist. It was never easy to make sure the information we were given was accurate. Employees' time cards by a time clock are an indicator, but not always a reliable one: a Chicago investigator found that of one hundred cards in one home thirty were blanks representing nothing but the operator's desire to fool the inspectors. We always asked to meet the RN supposed to be on duty at all times in some kinds of homes—and were told it was "her day off" many more times than the law of averages would suggest is possible. Sometimes, we learned, operators disguise their employees for an inspection by putting an RN cap on a practical nurse, or a practical nurse cap on an aide. Although it is often hard to find out just who is working there, it is easier to observe the dedication of the staff during a visit. Anyone can see whether most of the staff is working with the patients—or drinking coffee in the staff kitchen or watching television.

Beds are usually made promptly, with clean spreads, even in the worst-run of nursing homes. We learned to lift the spread to see if the sheets were clean as well—or if indeed there were any sheets at all. We looked in the linen closets to see if the supply of sheets, pillowcases, and towels seemed to be adequate for the number of patients. I was struck by how few blankets I saw on beds or in closets; some of the recurring nursing home horror stories are about patients shivering without blankets in the dead of winter. We visited the home's laundry to see how and by whom—sometimes by patients—the washing was done. In one home, we saw the owner washing sheets by hand and hanging them to dry by the furnace.

Many homes claim they have rehabilitation facilities. We visited a nationally known center for post-hospital rehabilitation, the Highland View Hospital in Cleveland. We saw there what rehabilitation should be—and we never saw anything remotely resembling it in any nursing home. At Highland View, each patient had a program of physical activity tailored to his individual need. The hospital equipment was outstanding, including even toilets specially made for paralyzed patients, and more important, the equipment was actually being used. Some patients were working at tasks they could handle and that would aid their rehabilitation. Although we have seen patients working in nursing homes, the purpose there was not to rehabilitate but to exploit: the only value of the patients' work was to save money for the owner.

Expensive rehabilitation equipment is now found in many nursing homes, if only because it is needed if the home is to qualify for Medicare. We found it well to determine if the equipment was being used—and discovered all too often that it was not, having been bought apparently only because someone else would pay for it. Idle equipment, gathering dust at government expense while the patients go without its benefits, gives all too accurate an indication of what is happening in most nursing homes. Even when the home had a physical therapist on the payroll, he often was little used because, as several therapists told us, the aides would not bother to bring the patients to them. We heard the same complaint from activities directors: the patients were not brought to them.

Food is, of course, a crucial part of the quality of nursing home life, and in most homes the timing of meals is as questionable as their quality. In order to save money on staff, the typical owner crams all three meals into one shift, feeding the patients at 8:00 A.M., 11:00 to 11:30, and 4:00 to 5:00 in the afternoon. (Indeed, in order to get them out of the way, patients are put to bed in some homes at 5:30.) As to the quality of the food, we quickly learned to compare the posted menus with what actually appeared at mealtimes. We examined the trays waiting on carts in kitchens and hallways. In most cases, they compared unfavorably with hospital food trays. While nursing homes typically used the same plastic dish with dividers, it was rare in the nursing home to see any utensil other than a spoon, rare to see bread and butter, rare to see juice, and when there was coffee, rare to find it accompanied by cream and sugar. Some homes had insulation to keep the food warm during the long time it took to distribute the trays, but most did not. We often saw food that should have been refrigerated, like salads, left out for hours before it was to be served. The cook in one hot kitchen we visited had installed fans that blew on the salads while they were waiting for mealtime.

We would ask if the home employed a dietitian—though I have never actually seen one. We counted chairs in the dining room and compared the total to the number of patients, to determine if an effort was made to help those patients who were able to leave their rooms at mealtimes to get to the dining room. We also watched during meals to see how much help patients were getting from the staff.

Refrigerators and freezers are good places to study the quality of nursing home food. We saw many refrigerators packed with big loaves of cheap, soft bread, and we were told that day-old bread is better for the patients—just as it is better, of course, for the owner's budget. We saw freezers with little in them except small packages wrapped in brown paper, which we were informed was meat; inspectors further informed us that much nursing home meat is in fact taken home by the owners.

We often asked how patients were fed during the long interval between dinner in the afternoon and breakfast the next morning. Invariably we were told that "nourishment," as it was always called, was provided before bedtime. Sometimes in the form of crackers, in other cases juice. We became skeptical in several homes when we compared the number of patients to the few cans of juice on the pantry shelves.

Emergency exits are clearly essential for a building that houses many people who cannot move easily or fast. We looked for the exits and fire escapes, and for the evacuation plan that is supposed to be posted in the home. Having seer these, however, we learned to be skeptical about their meaning. Many homes lock the exits to keep patients from wandering out; one home provided the fire department with keys to its locked exit doors. This means the patients' lives depend on what the staff does in case of fire. Evacuation plans have little meaning unless the staff knows what to do in an emergency, and given the high turnover in nursing home employment, any training given the staff today will largely be lost a few months hence. One administrator proudly pulled the alarm to demonstrate his evacuation plan to us—and no one in the whole place moved in response to the alarm. Most homes are required to have fire doors, and under some circumstances, a sprinkler system. Yet even sprinklers set into the ceilings are not a complete guarantee of a sprinkler system. One owner showed me the sprinklers, then admitted that he had never gone to the expense of putting in the pipes necessary to connect the sprinklers to the water supply—they were there only to fool the inspectors.

The three of us became adept at measuring the physical details of a nursing home: whether the halls and doors were wide enough for wheelchairs and beds to be moved through them—in many homes it was impossible to get a wheelchair into the bathroom and in some it could not be gotten around the beds—and whether the halls were equipped with railings, and the bathrooms with lifts for tubs and handrails for toilets. A great many homes we saw did not even have soap and toilet paper in their bathrooms.

Night, some inspectors say, is the time of truth in a nursing home. So one night we spent the hours from midnight to dawn moving around the floors of a large nursing home that had once been a hotel. About 3:00 A.M. we followed the night administrator as he hurried to a patient who was gasping in distress. The administrator told an aide to bring him the aspirator, but when the machine arrived it proved to be unusable for the simplest of reasons: the cord was too short to reach an outlet. With considerable effort, the patient and bed were moved to an outlet. But the aspirator still would not work, at which point the administrator discovered a part was missing. He sent an aide to call a police ambulance that would take the patient, still gasping for breath, to a hospital.

While that was going on, another aide was solving an image problem. The patient was clothed in a filthy gray gown, not proper hospital dress. Looking around the ward, the aide found a patient whose gown was comparatively clean. Shaking him awake, she stripped him of the clean gown and put it on the patient waiting for the ambulance. When the police arrived, they said the hospital would not

accept the patient unless the registered nurse in charge declared it was an "emergency." There was no RN on the premises (doubtless it was "her day off"), but the administrator
produced a practical nurse wearing an RN-style cap whose
statement of emergency the police were willing to accept.
Upon leaving, the police found their cot-stretcher would not
fit into the elevator of the seven-story building, so they had
to remove the patient from the stretcher and strap him into
a chair.

During the quieter hours of this particular night, several
of the aides told us that they held down full-time day jobs
besides working 11:00 P.M. to 7:00 A.M. in the home. Then, at
5:00 A.M., the aides went around the wards yelling to arouse
the patients, although it was three hours before breakfast.
They told us this was for the convenience of the daytime
staff, who would not be able to get breakfast served at 8:00
A.M. (and therefore fit all three meals into one shift) unless
the night employees took care of getting the patients up. This
sort of thing happens in hospitals also, to be sure; but the average stay in a nursing home is three years—usually the last
years of a person's life.

We pried as deeply as we could into the economics of
the homes we visited. We asked who owned the home-often,
as we shall see in later chapters, a difficult question to answer. We asked how many patients were supported by Medicaid and how many by Medicare. When we requested the
rates paid by private patients, we found that these were frequently accompanied by a wide range of extra charges, many
of which could be imposed practically at will by the administrator. As example, witness the schedule, pages 15-16,
which lists the remarkable number of "additional charges"
levied by the Fairfax Nursing Home, in Fairfax, Virginia, as
of 1967.* These extras came on top of basic monthly charges

---

* This sort of document is hard to come by, and I was unable to obtain a
more recent example. However, it clearly seems safe to assume, in this
specific case and in general, that conditions have *not* since improved.

that ranged, at that time, from $375 in a four-bed ward to $595 in a private room.

FAIRFAX NURSING HOME
Additional Charges

Admission sets	$ 3.50
Air Matress	45.00 per month
Air Worms	3.50
Alcohol	.50 per pint
Aspirator	5.00 per day or use
Baby Oil	1.00
Bed sore Care	3.00 per day
Bibs, Plastic	2.50
Bladder Irrigation Tray	1.50
Body Lotion	1.00
Catheters (Foley)	3.50
Catheterization Sets	2.00
Chest Restraints	10.00
Denture Cups	.25
Diabetic Diet	15.00 per month
Disposable Chux	.15 each
Dainage bags and tubing for Catheterization Sets	1.00
Emesis Basin	1.50
Enemas: Fleat/Oil	1.00
Foam Cusion or ring	4.85
Guest Trays:	
Luncheon or Breakfast	1.00
Evening Meal	1.50
Hand Feeding	45.00 per month
Hand restraints	3.00
Hypodermyclysis Sets	2.00
Intravenous Sets	2.00
Incontinent Care (including Chux)	80.00 per month
Intensive Nursing Care Terrace Floor	90.00 per month
Irrigation Set	1.50
Levin tubes	2.00

Liter Cytol Urologic Irrigating Fluid	2.50	—1 liter
Medicated powder	1.40	
Nasal Catheters	1.00	
Oxygen		
¼ tank or less	10.00	
½ tank	15.00	
Full tank	20.00	
Oxygen mask	1.00	
Personal laundry	10.00	per month
Plastic gloves	.10	
Posey Restraints	6.00	
Rectal tubes	1.00	
Restraining chair	N/C	
Shampoo	1.00	per pint
Sheepskin (Synthetic)	10.00	
Solutions for Clysis & I.V.'s	5.00	per bottle
Spray deodorant	1.30	
Suction machine	25.00	per month
Suction tube	.50	
Television in room	21.00	per room
Tissues	.25	
Trapeze	15.00	per month
Tube feeding	30.00	
Rubber Pants	5.00	
Walkers	3.00	
Wheel Chairs	15.00	per month
Senile care	90.00	per month
Syringes	1.00	

A fact sheet issued for families of prospective clients of the Fairfax home assured them that, for these rates, "your loved one will receive the finest in nursing home care." They were also told that, through Medicare, "your loved one may be entitled to receive up to 100 days care which is mostly paid for by the government." Then came the list of "additional charges" reproduced here. As can be seen, the only item on the list for which there is no charge is a "restraining chair," while a wheelchair may be had for an additional $15 per month. To sleep on an air mattress costs a patient an additional $45 per month; and if he develops bedsores (usually because of staff neglect), he has to pay an extra $3 per day for the treatment of them. An especially notable item is the $90 monthly extra charge for "senile care": the judgment as to whether or not a patient needs such care is made at the discretion of the administrator. In short, the opportunities for profit in this list are legion—and that the Fairfax list is not uncommon is indicated by the 1972 federal booklet on nursing home care, which advises people shopping for a nursing home to be sure to check on the extra charges.

More important than anything else we saw or heard was the evidence that the patients themselves presented. Much could be learned from observing their general appearance: whether they looked clean and well-groomed, how they and the staff responded to each other. We did riot expect miracles; a nursing home is not by nature a happy place. Still, we learned to tell the difference between people suffering unavoidably from age and illness and patients who were also suffering needlessly from the cruelty or indifference of those who were supposed to care for them.

Whenever possible, we spoke to patients. Those who could—and would—talk to us gave us sharp and accurate appraisals of the institutions that housed them. Some patients could not talk to us because they were senile or too ill or too discouraged. But there were other grim reasons for patient silence. Some were silent because they feared the staff; a few told us they would be punished if they criticized the home. Others were silent for another reason. They sat vacant-eyed, responding to nothing—because they had been drugged into oblivion, to keep them quiet for the convenience of the management. That silence is hard for me to forget.

Although I was visiting nursing homes as an observer, I could not help being at times a participant. Seeing in me a sympathetic outsider, patients or their relatives would call on me for help against the system in which they were trapped. I could not say no, so over the years I have been frequently drawn into the lives of individual patients. One case was that of John Stua.

John Stua was a blue-collar worker, a widower who, in his mid-fifties, had been crippled in a fall. He could walk only with a crutch and orthopedic shoes. Unable to work, he was forced to go on welfare. A second illness sent him back to the hospital, and when he was discharged, the hospital physician found him to be in good condition and recommended that he be returned to a boardinghouse. But because he was on welfare, the doctor's recommendation had to go through the hospital's social service department—and that is when the nursing home system got hold of John Stua.

The hospital social worker ignored the doctor's recommendation that he go to a boardinghouse. Instead, although his record read: "Discharged to Robb's Boarding House," she shipped him to a nursing home, where he was placed in a cottage. Upon his arrival, he was allegedly examined by the physician on call for that nursing home. Where the hospital doctor had found Stua in good condition, the house doctor, a few hours later, found him to be in need of maximum skilled nursing care—a diagnosis that entitled the nursing home to receive the maximum reimbursement rate from the state.

John Stua was a good catch for the nursing home. With his crutch and his orthopedic shoes, he could get around without assistance. In good health, he needed little care, while the home could collect from the state at the maximum-care rate. The only trouble with John Stua, from the management's point of view, was that he was strong-willed enough to carry on a long, and ultimately successful, struggle for freedom.

While he was there, John Stua kept a diary in which he recorded the details of nursing home life. I was later to see that diary and find that it accorded with my own observation of that home. Here arc some excerpts;

"Feb. 7. Dinner—1 ½ plum, 2. B. coffee, like tea. 2. bread, ½ bowl soup. Dale said it was stew, but the woman put water in it. He is a liar. It was no stew in the first place, 1 gal. can for all. (I seen it). . . . Feb. 15, 6:20 A.M.—1 spoon scramble powder egg. 2 bread, 2 peces peaches. Lousy hamburger size of 50¢ pece. . . ."

On February 16 Stua commented on an article that had appeared in the Cleveland Press: "4600 in nursing homes. 2000 on Welfare. Not to increase money but increase food and allowance and supervise by qualified nurses and DR. *Not* by any Tom and Harry." Two days later: "I wonder how egg and bacon taste or soup without sugar. Hungry every day. . . ."

The weeks advanced. March 27: "It's lousy, I'm hungry, no money. . . . . I get at the most $10 of food a month and what I get is rotten. Their crooks and stealers . . ." Then, one day, he prints in all capital letters: "BEST MEAL I HAD. . . .D—ll:4O A.M.—HONEST TO GOD THE BEST IN ONE YEAR. HAM. PEAS. SWEET POTATOES. BREAD. COFFEE." On April 3, he writes: "My $5 aid not received and for six or 7 mo." (He is referring to the so-called "personal expense money" of five dollars, which he is supposed to receive monthly out of his welfare check.) And then he adds: "My eyeglasses are gone for a week."

April 6: "No one will help me to get the hell out . . . Howard thru a cigarette in the wast basket and almost started a fire. Smoke the dump all up. The fire drill is marked. And it a lie, not one fire drill since I here . . ."

A holiday note: "Easter day in the nut house. I hope the family that own this dump see no more Easter."

In May Stua wrote: "I ask the nurse for a smoke. She said don't have any. No check. No smoke. No eat." Then he added the note that represents the first step toward his freedom: "Wrote a letter today." But, he noted later, "no answer comes," so on June i: "Letter I mail today to Mrs. Ludwig." (Mrs. Ludwig was a city nurse.) Twice again in early July he reports writing further appeals, but "no one come." Then on July 15 he wrote: "Two women came to see me about this rat hole."

The two women were Patricia Kelley, who had accompanied me on many nursing home visits, and myself. We were there because I had, through a roundabout route, obtained a copy of the first letter John Stua had written, to the Secretary of Health, Education, and Welfare in Washington. We went to check on what he had said. Although we could do little, if anything, for John Stua, the very fact of our presence was a threat to the home's operators—a brother and sister, the sister being the registered nurse required by regulations.

Our questions appeared to catch them somewhat off balance. We asked who had decided, contrary to the hospital recommendation, that Stua needed skilled nursing home care. When they said the nursing home physician had found him to be "combative, abusive, mentally deranged," we asked to see the diagnosis. We were told that, on that very day, the physician had taken all the patients' records back to his office. When we asked if it was true that Stua was not receiving his monthly allowance for personal expenses, the brother-operator held up a new five-dollar bill. We were told that they had withheld the allowance—just for this month—because of Stua's alcoholic tendencies. (In fact, there was no report of alcoholism in his prenursing home medical record. If he were an alcoholic, he could not have maintained much of a habit on five dollars a month.) And because Stua was mentally ill, the operators told us, they had just arranged with his caseworker to have him transferred to another nursing home that handled "mild mental" patients.

We then went to the cottage to talk to John Stua. We found him sitting, rigid and angry, on the side of his bed. His clean white sports shirt, clean slacks, and socks, all of which he had washed himself, showed he cared about his personal appearance. He told his story rapidly and intently—and he sounded entirely rational to us. He brought forth his diary from a footlocker under his bed and showed it to me. We checked his allegations item by item, and found them accurate. The evening meal was served at the time he had recorded, and the quality was as low as his description. His eyeglasses were missing, his dentures obviously needed repair, and his orthopedic shoes were badly worn—he was entitled to services remedying all of these, and had received none of them.

Our visit had a surprising outcome. The next day, instead of sending him to the "mild mental" nursing home, the operators packed John Stua and his belongings in a taxi and shipped him to the county welfare office, and from there he went back to a boardinghouse in his old neighborhood.

John Stua's story is unusual only because the system was beaten, and that happened because we outsiders opened the door of that nursing home and looked at what was going on inside. In other respects his story is all too typical—notably in the operators' practice of charging the government the maximum rate for someone who only needs minimum care, and then not delivering even that minimum. John Stua happened to be a welfare patient in a profit-making home, but the abuse of nursing home patients is not restricted to those circumstances. I have investigated cases of private patients in nonprofit homes who were treated just as badly as was John Stua.

Patients like John Stua—the one million Americans in nursing homes—are what this book is ultimately about, although it may not always seem that way in the chapters that follow. Those chapters deal with the financial manipulations of profit-hungry nursing home operators and the corruption of government regulators who allow the operators to have their way with the public's money. There is a kind of dark humor in the accounts that appear in this book. We cannot help chuckling at the utter dedication of the swindling nursing home operator as he assiduously invents new ways to pick our pockets and line his own—but it is the patient who pays the bill in human suffering. We may smile at the operator who thought of putting in sprinklers without pipes, but the smile fades when we read that ten—or fifty-patients died in yesterday's nursing home fire. And there is no humor at all if you pay a visit to the morgue, as I have often done, to check with the coroner on the condition of bodies that come from nursing homes—a grim but effective way to evaluate the treatment those people got there. Behind the thievery and the corruption that this book describes is the physical reality of the stinking nursing homes in which our old people are dying a living death—and that is why, above all, the swindling should matter to us.

IN THE FIRST YEARS, as I came to see the sad reality of nursing home life in my own state, I was led to believe that conditions might be better outside Ohio. Much of what was wrong was blamed on systems of regulation and the methods by which government, the biggest buyer of nursing home services, paid the operators. Other states practiced different methods, and it was possible to hope that they got better results. I went to see for myself, and I have by now visited more than two hundred nursing homes around the country and interviewed countless officials in twenty-one states ranging from Hawaii and Alaska to Massachusetts and Florida.

But sad to say, it is the same everywhere. All over the country, nursing homes are similar, and similarly bad. Excellent homes are rare, and most of those that are considered good are good only by comparison to the majority that are worse. Some states pay twice as much as others for nursing home patients, but the extra cost does not buy better care. Reimbursement methods and regulations vary greatly from state to state without, however, producing any material difference in how the patients are treated.

It disturbs me, as it will others, that I seem to tar all nursing homes with one sweep of the brush. Of the more than two hundred homes I have personally seen, I could honestly call only one a good home. In that home, I felt that an honest attempt at good care was being made by those in charge, despite the limited knowledge we have about treatment of elderly people. Perhaps it was the fact that the personnel admitted areas of failure, that they showed me things they considered wrong, that encouraged me the most. What I saw I liked, and what I heard I believed. This home happened to be a church-sponsored home—but I have seen other church-sponsored homes that are dreadful. This home charged high rates—but I have seen more expensive homes that delivered very poor care.

The industry's response to the charges in this book is predictable. Its representatives will surely point out that I have visited only a small fraction of the nation's nearly 23,000 nursing homes* and therefore cannot generalize from what I have seen. They will say that anything I have found—whether it be patient abuse or financial manipulation—is an "isolated instance." The industry is likely also to say that I am damaging its public image and that problems in the nursing homes, if indeed there are any problems, should be resolved by the industry itself. That was the gist of a couple of hours of monologue delivered to me in 1969 by Donald W. Gormly, past president of the California Nursing Home Association and treasurer of the national association. Two years later Gormly, his wife, and his ac-

---

* The estimate of the Department of Health, Education, and Welfare. These are divided into three categories, according to the amount of medical care they are supposed to provide. In descending order of amount of care, there are 4,057 Extended Care Facilities licensed to receive Medicare payments, 6,500 Skilled Nursing Homes and 12,000 Intermediate Care Facilities, the latter two both being licensed to receive Medicaid payments. In this book the term "nursing home" is used to describe all three categories.

countant were indicted on a charge of fraudulently padding the bills paid by the state and federal government for patients in one of the Gormly nursing homes—the prosecutor said the amount involved might run as high as $3 million—and in March 1972 Gormly was convicted on charges of conspiracy, filing false reports, and grand theft. He was fined $5,000, placed on five-year probation, and required to return $1.2 million to the state. In retrospect, it was not surprising that Mr. Gormly wanted the industry to be allowed to police itself.

Too much evidence has been accumulated from too many sources for the industry to be able to sustain its case that the result of any one investigation is no more than "isolated instances." It is true that no one investigator, whether private or official, has gone into all 23,000 homes—but it is also true that repeated investigations, whether of 10 homes or 50 or 200, have all painted equally dismal pictures of poor patient care and financial manipulations by owners. Of all the regulatory officials I have met, not one told me that only a minority of the homes under his jurisdiction were unsatisfactory.

Every few months a fragment of the truth appears in the press: a local expose of brutal treatment of patients, or most tragically, still another fire that kills a dozen or more patients, in a home known to have been in violation of fire regulations. In early 1971 the Chicago *Tribune* ran a hair-raising series by reporters who had gotten jobs in a dozen nursing homes in that city. They reported dreadful patient abuse by owners who, it was later learned, were getting rich at the expense of their victims.

Large-scale exposés have also been made. In 1971 a group of Nader's Raiders headed by Claire Townsend published, under the title *Old Age: The Last Segregation,* a description of what they found in twenty-three nursing homes in the East. My own investigation in Cleveland, submitted to the Senate Subcommittee on Long-Term Care, was sent on to the General Accounting Office. The GAO sent a team of six investigators to Cleveland. They confirmed my findings, which the subcommittee had called "the most detailed available account of nursing home abuses in any one city." Since then detailed accounts of abuses in other cities and states have become available.

The Senate Subcommittee on Long-Term Care has held a total of twenty-nine hearings on nursing homes in the last decade. Hearings held in Boston, Chicago, and Minneapolis proved especially fruitful, turning up a wealth of information on patient abuse and owner profiteering. And this is not the only congressional committee to report what is happening in the nursing home industry. The Senate Finance Committee, in its 1969 hearings, heard testimony that nursing home owners and their allies, notably physicians and pharmacists, were exploiting the government's Medicare and Medicaid programs. This is some of what the Committee staff learned:

> Unnecessary services are being provided on a widespread basis in nursing homes. . . . The majority of the extended care facilities [nursing homes licensed for Medicare] participating in the program do not fully meet the standards set in the law and regulations . . . Evidence exists that "kick back" arrangements between suppliers—such as pharmacies and physical therapists—and nursing homes may be widespread. . . . There is substantial evidence that many physicians are engaging in the practice known as "gang visits" to nursing home and hospital patients. Under this practice a physician may see as many as 30, 40 and 50 patients in a day in the same facility—regardless of whether the visit is medically necessary or whether any service is actually furnished. . . . Another cause for concern is the alarming growth in chain operations in the nursing home field. Some of these chains actively solicit physician purchase of stock to assure a high occupancy rate. Other chains purchase stock of hospital supply and pharmaceutical supply houses. This leads to arrangements

with respect to intercompany sales at what may very well be higher than would otherwise be paid—a form of captive market used to milk the Medicare trust funds. . . . We have found inflated depreciation allowances and many sales of facilities at inflated prices in order to get maximum payments from Medicare.

Support for at least some of the Senate Finance Committee's conclusions can be found in the reports of the General Accounting Office. In addition to its Ohio investigation, which resulted from the information we had turned up in Cleveland, the GAO has reported on financial irregularities in nursing homes in five other states—Oklahoma, Michigan, California, New York, and Connecticut—and at this writing, is investigating nursing homes in Tennessee, Massachusetts, and Colorado. Two of those states, California and New York, have conducted their own investigations of their Medicaid programs; they turned up evidence of widespread looting of government money by the nursing homes.

Certainly regulatory officials in the many states I visited did not think their problems consisted only of "isolated instances." On the contrary, they all held that poor patient care and financial manipulation were major problems in the nursing homes in their respective states. Certainly the National Council of Senior Citizens would not agree that patient abuse consists of isolated instances. Nor would former Congressman David Pryor of Arkansas. Congressman Pryor became a crusader for nursing home reform after he worked as an aide in an institution near Washington. After he had spoken out on the subject, people all over the nation—patients, relatives, employees, even state officials—began sending Pryor their complaints about the quality of nursing home care. By the time I interviewed him in 1971, Pryor's files held many thousands of such complaints from every state in the country; each state provided at least one bulging manila folder of complaints. Finally, if all were well in the industry, it does not seem likely that the President of the United States would have devoted a major address, in 1971, to the need for nursing home reform.

Many people not concerned about the industry as a whole will contend that they have found good nursing homes for their relatives. They may have done so. Different factors, of course, go into the making of such an evaluation: the frequency, or lack of it, of visits to the home, the times at which visits are made, the physical and mental infirmity of the patient, the family's expectations about the home. Sometimes such favorable views may be at least partly attributable to people's guilt feelings about having used a nursing home to dispose of an unwanted relative. Few of us, at any rate, have the courage to see what we do not want to see.

The operators themselves testify to the generally low quality of care. As I learned at the very start, many nursing home operators are prone to deplore what happens in other homes while praising their own enterprise. In this situation, carried to its extreme, each home is thus being criticized by another, leaving none unscathed. But my purpose is not to describe the quality of care provided in each home in the country. Enough homes furnish poor care to worry all sensitive Americans, and each American is likely to have a brush with a nursing home in some form. If he escapes placing a relative in a home, he may end up in a home himself. While he awaits his turn, he is paying taxes to support nursing homes for others—and each year the cost rises, as do his taxes. As a result, no one can afford to ignore the nursing home crisis. Unwittingly, we are all caught in it, even though we may think we have placed a relative in a good home. Each of us has every reason to be concerned not only with the quality of care but with the reasons for the quality of that care, if it is low.

Bad nursing homes seem to be contagious. If enough homes in an area provide poor care, the other homes in the area tend also to decline. And when there is no good place to which a concerned family can move a patient, the incentive for a home to deliver quality care at fair rates is destroyed. One has only to have had a relative in a nursing home to understand this tragic snowballing of neglect. Complaints are frequently met with the chilling brush-off, "If you don't like it here, take your mother someplace else." If there is no place better to take her, there is no reason for that home to improve.

These realities give the lie to the operators' standard line: Give us more money and we'll deliver better care. Their case was stated most memorably by Saul Tobias, a Massachusetts operator testifying before the Senate Sub-committee on Long-Term Care in Boston. Tobias compared the situation of the nursing home to that of a vending machine: "The nursing home is the vending machine; the welfare department is the customer. If the customer wants the ten-cent bar and puts in a nickel, don't bang the vending machine. It gave what it got."

Tobias's metaphor is a good one, for all too often the nursing home industry does behave like a vending machine. All that's wrong with his statement is the numbers. It would be more accurate to say that government is putting in ten cents for the nickel bar, and not always getting even that; furthermore, if the operators continue to be successful in lobbying for higher rates, soon the taxpayers will be paying a quarter for that same nickel bar. (There is an ironic sidelight to the image of the nursing home as vending machine. Almost every home I have visited actually has at least one such machine, and often I have watched patients putting in their coins for candy or cigarettes. Many times, far more often than seems the case with machines elsewhere, I have watched the patient feebly bang the machine, and get nothing, not even his money back.)

Nor does the standard line of most nursing home critics —more regulation will produce better care—make sense in the light of nursing home realities. State and federal governments have elaborate regulations governing nursing homes, but those regulations remain unenforced at all levels of government, and for good reason: there is no will to enforce, and a lot of money to be made by nonenforcement. As long as that will is lacking, new regulations will only lull the public with the illusion of progress. The director of Aid for the Aged in Cuyahoga County had been right when, at the beginning of my investigation, he warned me against the twin illusions of more money and more regulations.

One conclusion is inescapable: nursing homes are a very lucrative business. Despite the pleas of poverty from operators caught cutting corners in the care of their patients, despite the chorus demanding higher government payments, despite the many variations I have heard on the theme of Saul Tobias and his vending machine—give us a dime and we'll give you a dime's worth of service—it became abundantly clear to me that nursing home operators are getting rich at the expense of their patients and the taxpayer.

The evidence comes in many forms. It is in the countless frauds perpetrated by the nursing home operators: the patients cheated of the few dollars they are entitled to call their own; the government charged for medical services never delivered, for drugs that never reached the patient, for equipment unneeded and never used. These frauds, each of them petty in themselves, add up to unknown millions of dollars a year. The evidence is in the moneylenders who have gone into the nursing home industry, men like Joseph Kosow of Boston, who lend nursing homes mortgage money at up to 40 percent interest a year—interest rates ultimately paid for by the public. And the evidence was in the 1968-1970 boom in nursing home stocks, which led a new-issue underwriter to observe: "Nobody can lose money in this business. There's just no way."

The evidence also takes oblique form in the Cadillacs in which the operators travel. Not long ago, at a meeting of nursing home operators called by the Connecticut Department of Welfare (the purpose of which, incidentally, was for the operators to plead their case for higher government reimbursement rates), an official noticed an unusual number of Cadillacs in the parking lot. He checked the plates with the Motor Vehicle Department and found that nineteen of the twenty-three Cadillacs belonged to nursing home operators. The same general message has often been stated to me by Sanford Novak, the first operator I met. When I run into him, Sandy is fond of saying: "Stick with me, Mary Adelaide, and you'll be driving a Caddie, too."

More systematic evidence of the profit in nursing homes is now available. Because of the growing belief that the operators were making more out of their government revenue than they cared to admit, the Federation for Community Planning of Cleveland commissioned a study of the cost of nursing home care by a respected consultant firm, GEOMET, Inc., of Rockville, Maryland. The consultant was to determine the average cost of nursing home care in a home meeting all state and federal requirements. Using 1970 figures for costs and the then Medicaid rate of $14 a day, the GEOMET study found that a hypothetical hundred-bed home in Cleveland would earn a 39 percent profit on each Medicaid patient.* That could mean an annual return on the owner's equity of as much as 76 percent. In other words, you could earn your investment back in less than two years. Comparable figures have come from other sources. In 1971 the Connecticut Hospital Commission calculated that the owner of a forty-bed nursing home in that state who had invested 25.0 percent of the value of the property could earn an annual return of 39.3 percent on his investment. In 1972 the General Accounting Office reportedly studied a sampling of homes in New York and concluded they were earning a 450 percent return in five years on their investment.

* The figures in greater detail arc as follows: The hypothetical home was built in 1966 at a cost of $442,843, plus $100,000 for equipment, for a total of $542,843. If the home is 92 percent occupied with Medicaid patients at $14 a day, the annual before-tax profit would be $183,682.

These are profits a defense contractor himself might envy. Yet even these figures understate what most operators can earn. For one thing, the GEOMET study assumed that each home conformed to all government regulations; but 36 percent of the homes in the study failed in varying degrees to so conform, and therefore their costs would be lower—and their profits higher.* For another, the study did not take into account profits based on fraud. Yet fraudulent practices in the industry are, to say the least, widespread and it is a safe assumption that a large proportion of operators are picking up some amount, large or small, on the side by one or more of the many easy ways of cheating the patients and the government—and not getting caught at it.

If an operator in Ohio can make 76 percent a year on his investment, in Connecticut 39 percent, and if some operators in New York can make 450 percent in five years, how about the rest of the country? Studies similar to those of GEOMET, the Connecticut Hospital Commission, and the GAO have not been made in other states. Ohio's Medicaid rate—and 60 percent of nursing home patients in this country are on Medicaid—is about the national average, and so are its costs. Some states with large numbers of nursing homes, like Massachusetts and New York, have much higher Medicaid rates, though the quality of care they deliver does not seem to be different. So it is fair to assume that operators in the nation as a whole do as well as they do in Ohio. And that means they are doing very well indeed.

As THE NURSING HOME BUSINESS has flourished, so has its advertising. In a suddenly brisk market, the nursing home

---

* Questioned about this high percentage of transgressors. Dr. John Cashman, director of the Ohio Department of Health, commented that his department knew that many inspectors did not do their job properly, and that too many homes were in violation—but what, he asked, did people want the department to do, turn 24,000 patients out into the street by closing all the homes that have violations?

business has turned to the Yellow Pages of telephone directories to take their story to potential buyers, following the
advice in a manual, published by the Attending Staff Association of Downey, California, called *Nursing Home Administration:*

> Advertise in the yellow pages. Your telephone directory is
> the first thing consulted by numbers of people whenever they
> face a need, whether for garden hose, a plasterer, or a home
> for the aged.

The manual suggests "happiness benefits" to be ac-
cented in the advertising: "Life is happy. . . ."; "The guest
is the center of everything. . . ."; "Freedom to live their own
lives . . ."; "Many special outings . . ."; "Beauty all around
them . . ."; "Singing canaries, with fish to match." Singing
fish are all right, but the manual sternly advises administrators not to go too far: "If there is no organ, do not lure customers with the hope of organ music."

Many Americans, especially those with any direct experience of a nursing home, are undoubtedly aware that the
industry's self-promotion bears little resemblance to the
dreary reality of those institutions in which we warehouse
our old people. But public awareness of the nursing home
problem is uneven. While many people seem to sense that
the quality of care is poor, far fewer seem to connect that
knowledge with the fact that this is a highly profitable industry inhabited by an unconscionable number of chiselers and
con men.

Documenting the ways in which nursing home profiteers
conduct their business has occupied virtually all my time in
the past few years, and the purpose of this book is to report
on what I have found. Only an informed public can force a
response from the government agencies responsible for nursing homes. What happens in our nursing homes is a public,
not a private, responsibility. It is government that places most
patients in nursing homes, government that supplies most of

the industry's income. So far government has offered us nothing more than promises in response to the sordid revelations about the nursing home industry. (The latest set of promises, made by President Nixon in August 1971, is described in Chapter 11.) After the experience of almost a decade, it is abundantly clear to me that, with honorable exceptions, there is no will in government to defend the helpless patients and the taxpayers' money that are in its charge. To understand why this is so, we must begin by understanding the large and complex role that government plays in the nursing home industry.

2

Government: Where the Money Comes From

THE NURSING HOME as a money-making enterprise is quite new in America. As recently as the 1930s there were only a handful of nursing homes in this country, and those few were mostly of the mom-and-pop type that is now disappearing. Larger homes were usually run on a nonprofit basis by a church or fraternal order as a service for their membership, or by local government as a "poor folks home." Most of these homes could never meet the legal specifications for nursing homes today, but many of them undoubtedly were better places for a patient to be than the average "modern" nursing home.

The industry began to grow in response to the great changes that became evident in America after the Second World War. As we all know, people are living longer: the number of Americans over sixty-five totaled over 20 million by 1973 and is rising by 300,000 to 400,000 each year. The number of older people who are sick but still alive has grown just as rapidly, so there has been a vast increase in the number of people who just cannot take care of themselves on their own.

In the past, a past that seems very distant now, older people were taken care of by their families. They lived out their last years in the homes of their grown children. That, too, has changed. Older people now live alone as long as they can, but for many that time ends long before the end of their lives. For many who are sick, who are alive but cannot manage alone, the only answer is the nursing home. And some go because they and their children reject each other.

They usually cannot pay for the nursing home they need, for the old are generally poor as well as sick: people over sixty-five have less than half the income of people under that age, although they need twice as much health care. Health insurance never covers long-term nursing home costs, and for a variety of reasons, the children of old people frequently will not pay for them. In addition, many old people have no responsible relatives; half the people in nursing homes have no immediate family at all. Other old people have drifted apart from their families; the children are living far away, or are indifferent, or both. Many families do care but cannot afford the cost of a nursing home for the parent—the bill now averages around $14 a day. Finally, even if they can pay, society no longer holds the children responsible for their parents. This change, in effect the end of the family unit, is now recognized by law, for, when the resources of the old are calculated, the income of their children is not included. The son may be making $100,000 a year and own a winter home in Florida, but if his mother has no income she qualifies for public housing or Medicaid or other forms of assistance to the poor. That seems to be the way we Americans want it to be. (When, in the 1972 election campaign, a New York newspaper revealed that the mother of Congress-woman Bella Abzug, a successful lawyer, was receiving Medicaid, the public reaction was in favor of the congress-woman.)

That leaves only the government. Americans have turned over the responsibility for older people, when they are sick and poor, to the state. What happens to old people is decided not by families but by bureaucracies, and the nurs-

ing home industry, though privately owned, is a government
industry much like the Lockheed Aircraft Corporation. By
1971 two-thirds of the million people in nursing homes were
supported by government, and more than three-quarters of
the $3.5 billion income of nursing homes was public mon-
ey.

The Social Security system, born in 1935, was the federal government's first major financial involvement with the
elderly. Although Social Security then provided no nursing
home money as such, it added to the amount available to pay
nursing home bills. In 1950, with an amendment to the Social
Security Act, Congress first provided that direct federal payments could be made to nursing homes, though the amount
was very small compared to what was to come later.

That first trickle was, however, enough to whet the appe-
tite, for some of the eminent hustlers described in later chapters of this book make their first appearance in the 1950s.
They were the first to see the exciting profit potential in the
nursing home, the first to view it as a business rather than as
a service or an occupation. The percentage of homes run for
profit has been rising ever since. The time of the hustlers had
arrived, and it is with us still. (I do not mean to imply that
the old mom-and-pop nursing home was paradise. Many of
those operators were incompetent, and others were brutal.
But they were not in the business because it was lucrative—
it wasn't in those days.)

Public money began flooding the health-care system, including nursing homes, after the adoption in 1965 of Medicare
and Medicaid. Medicare (Title XVIII of the Social Security
Act) provided federal financing for most forms of health care
for people over sixty-five years of age, regardless of income.
Included in that care is up to one hundred days in a nursing
home, provided that this follows hospitalization. Medicaid
(Title XIX), which is financed jointly by the federal and respective state governments, pays for health care for the poor of
any age. Medicaid will pay for an unlimited nursing home stay.

Those two acts set off a series of profound changes in the health industry, nowhere more than in nursing homes. Because they were conceived in illusion and born through political compromise, Medicare and Medicaid have cost far more and produced far less than their sponsors had hoped. Money was suddenly pumped into a system that had neither the capacity nor the desire to expand rapidly, with the result that much of the new money disappeared into higher costs rather than into more service for those who needed it. Health-care prices, including those for nursing homes, went up much faster than the general price level in the years after Medicare and Medicaid, and in the nursing home industry especially, the new programs as they were run became a guarantee of excess profits with no benefit to the patient.

The flaws in Medicare and Medicaid were not due to carelessness or ignorance but are, along with the continuing abuses of the programs, the results of the politics of health. When federally financed health insurance for the poor and the elderly was first suggested, it was vigorously opposed by the health-care establishment, notably the formidable American Medical Association and the American Hospital Association (though the members of those two organizations later turned out to be the chief beneficiaries of the new programs). Using the cry of socialized medicine, these organizations lobbied against anything that threatened their right to decide which patients needed what treatment and how much that treatment was worth. What did come out of the long struggle over federal health insurance were programs under which Washington poured money into the health industry with a minimum of regulation of how that money was used. In effect, the sponsors of Medicaid and Medicare said to the industry: "Let us give you the money, and we won't look too closely at how it's spent."

That fatal compromise is the root cause of the nursing home industry's ability to extract excess profits from the government. Once having taken on the responsibility for older Americans who are sick and poor, the government never exercised the will to ensure the proper carrying out of this responsibility by the institutions to which the old were entrusted. As we shall see repeatedly in the chapters that follow, the failure of government has been massive at all levels, from federal officials who administer their programs in such a way as to guarantee their ignorance of what is happening to the billions of dollars they spend, down to local inspectors and caseworkers who close their eyes to the abuses they see every day in the nursing homes. The patient lying abandoned in a urine-soaked bed, starved, abused at will by aides, is just as surely a victim of governmental indifference as of the greed of the owner.

In theory, there is an elaborate network of regulation to cover both Medicaid and Medicare. Briefly, this is how it is supposed to work in relation to nursing homes. Medicaid, by far the bigger source of money for nursing homes because it has no time limit, is regulated mainly by the states. Each state, usually through its health department, licenses and inspects nursing homes that take Medicaid patients; it is the inspector who decides whether the home is meeting state and federal standards. Each state also decides who is to be eligible for Medicaid. Medicaid was intended for the "medically indigent," those who cannot afford the care they need; the income limit varies from state to state, and is usually somewhat higher than the income limit on welfare. In this system, the local welfare caseworker plays an essential part. The caseworker decides whether an applicant is eligible for Medicaid, and if the applicant has some resources (Social Security, in most cases), how much more Medicaid should pay the nursing home for his care. Most important, it is the caseworker who usually chooses the nursing home for the Medicaid patient. Thus the nursing home operator is dependent on the inspector (who can close his home for violations) and the caseworker (who can either guarantee or close off his supply of patients). It is in these relationships that the corruption and indifference of nursing home regulators are most painfully evident.

The states also decide the rates that nursing homes are paid for Medicaid patients. There are two main ways of paying the Medicaid bill: (1) flat rate (the nursing home gets so much a day per patient, paid directly to the home) and (2) cost plus (the nursing home is reimbursed for its costs, plus a "reasonable" profit). Washington's role is mainly confined to paying the federal share of the cost, which ranges from 50 to 80 percent, depending on the state. Medicare, which pays for about 4 percent of the nursing home population, who are there for short stays after hospitalization, operates entirely on the cost-plus approach, and is 100 percent federally financed. These, however, are not the only ways in which federal money reaches the nursing home. If a patient gets Social Security, his Medicaid bill is reduced by that amount. The Veterans Administration also pays nursing homes for the care of patients coming out of VA hospitals. Some patients receive funds under federal programs like Old Age Assistance, and turn the checks over to the nursing home.

The advent of Medicaid and Medicare was a clear signal to those seeking a fast way to make money. Those businessmen and hustlers already in the industry saw the new money as a way to expand their operations and their profits. The industry expanded, and prices went up. The patients suffered, not so much because anyone set out to make them suffer (though that happens, too), but because the federal money included no incentives for improving patient care. Exactly the opposite was true: much of the operators' increased profits comes out of the hide of the patient.

Flat-rate Medicaid money is the most profitable to the operator, and the hardest on the patient. If the government will pay, say, $14 a day per patient, the way to make money is obviously to cut daily costs as far below $14 as you can. Some costs, like real estate taxes and interest, cannot be cut;

so, since most of those which can be lowered have to do with patient care, that is where the operator cuts corners. First of all, you buy cheap food in the smallest possible amounts: operators have been found, in the 1970s, to be feeding patients on less than $1.00 a day, and one, in Chicago in 1970, managed to feed his patients on $.78 a day.* Not surprisingly, many nursing home patients are emaciated. You can also cut corners on staff. Hire a cheaper practical nurse instead of a registered nurse; for aides, pay the lowest rate and get people who can't hold a job anywhere else. The patients will suffer—much of the brutality in nursing homes comes from incompetent aides who seem to be taking out their own inadequacies on the people in their charge—but the profits will go up. These variable costs are those parts of the nursing home operation that on paper are the most subject to governmental regulation—so, if the operator can cut those costs, it is because the regulators let him get away with it. From the point of view of the operator, it is cheaper to buy off an inspector or caseworker than to pay the cost of decent patient care.

In a flat-rate system, healthy patients are desirable. John Stua, described in Chapter 1, was such a patient. The operator gets the same $14 a day whatever the amount spent on care of the patient, so the less care the patient needs, the higher the profit margin on the $14. The result is that an astonishing number of the people in nursing homes should not be there at all. Every critical student of nursing homes has come to that conclusion; they vary only on the percentage of healthy patients. The General Accounting Office, after studying a sample of patients in Michigan, con-

---

* As late as October 1973, after the year's great increase in food prices, the state of New York charged that a Brooklyn nursing home was feeding its patients for $.30 a meal. This establishment, the Liberty Nursing Home, had also diverted money from patients' personal allowances, the state inspectors said. They concluded that Medicaid since 1968 had paid Liberty more than $2.5 million for patient care, "although far less than this amount has been received in services."

cluded that almost 80 percent (297 out of 378) did not require skilled nursing care.* A 1971 study of New York City Medicaid patients in nursing homes, by the state comptroller's office, found that from 53 to 61 percent of the patients did not need to be there. Daphne Krause, of the Minneapolis Age and Opportunity Center, which has studied homes in that area, gave a figure of 30 to 40 percent. In Cleveland, the head of the nursing home Medicaid program put the proportion of patients unnecessarily in homes under her jurisdiction at 90 percent.

Some of my saddest experiences have been with patients who were healthy and wanted to get out of the nursing home—but couldn't. (Legally, of course, the patient is free to leave. But that legal right means little to a person who is old and cut off from the world, without money to tide him over till the next Social Security check, without relatives, without even access to a telephone. If, as typically happens, the caseworker refuses to help, the chances of getting out are further diminished.) It should be noted that this does not mean all those people could go home and live alone. Some undoubtedly could, but many, perhaps most, need the custodial care of a rest home, or so-called "intermediate care facility." Such care costs substantially less than that in a "skilled nursing home," which, at least in theory, provides skilled nursing care around the clock.

Healthy patients are in nursing homes for a variety of reasons. Some originally needed to be there, after a stay in a hospital, but while they are recovered now, neither the operator nor anyone else makes a move to discharge them. The operator keeps them for profit, and no one else seems to care. Some are there because the caseworker was lazy, or careless, or wanted to do a favor for the nursing home operator, who had an empty bed. Or the favor, for a healthy or not-so-healthy patient, may come from a friendly physician—

* Through use of older, and less strict, criteria this figure was subsequently revised downward to "only" 42 percent.

as long ago as 1961, when the Attending Staff Association of Downey, California, published its manual, *Nursing Home Administration,* in which administrators were advised: "If a doctor likes you and believes in you, he may send you enough patients to keep you fully occupied. A telephone call to let him know when you have a vacancy may be all that you need to do." The Four Seasons nursing home chain made the relationship more direct: when the chain was going to build a nursing home in a community, it got local doctors to invest in the operation, so their referrals would add to the return on their own investment.

Collusion between caseworkers and doctors and nursing homes is often rumored, but government has shown no interest in investigating the subject, although the potential savings to the taxpayer would be great if some of the healthy patients could be discharged or moved to less expensive institutions. The GAO, in its Ohio investigation, decided the subject was beyond its scope, and contented itself with the observation that "it is conceivable that the nursing home operator may find it beneficial to pay welfare workers for referring to his home patients who are in need of little care, or to seek cooperative arrangements with physicians designed to secure patients needing little care."

The patients seldom object, though occasionally a healthy person in a nursing home fights for his freedom. It takes a lot of courage to fight in that setting, and few of us have it. The tragedy is that he may not stay healthy long. The typical nursing home is not an environment that encourages recovery; if it is not damaging to his health, it certainly saps his will to live and take care of himself. Soon he becomes physically, or more likely mentally, unable to cope. Then he does need the nursing home he did not need when he came.

The game of profit is played differently in those situations where the nursing home is paid, not a flat rate per patient day, but by reimbursement of its costs. This is the method used by Medicare, and in some states by Medicaid also. There is no incentive to cut costs in this situation, since the costs are passed on to the government. The opportunity for the operator in this case lies in padding his bills, which is made easy by the fact that government rarely conducts any effective audit of nursing home bills.

The extra (or "ancillary") services that government purchases for nursing home patients provide another rich field for exploitation. The opportunity for profit here lies in the operator's relationship with people for whose goods and services the government pays. Although the operator does not collect the money—it is paid directly to the supplier—he has the power to determine who will, since it is he who chooses the suppliers and decides how much the supplier has to deliver. Thus the operator decides which pharmacist will get the considerable drug business his home provides, and since he cannot demand a lower price, because the government is paying, it is common practice for him to demand a kickback from the pharmacist he docs choose. And, as we shall see in Chapter 8, if the operator is at all unscrupulous, he has other opportunities to make extra money with the pharmacist. He can order expensive brand-name drugs and let the pharmacist fill the prescription with much cheaper generic drugs that are identical to the brand-name drugs; the government pays the higher price and the operator and pharmacist split the difference. Or he can order drugs in unnecessarily large quantities. Or—most simply and with the greatest profit— bill the government for drugs that are never delivered at all. There is a melancholy sidelight to the drug business in nursing homes. As anyone who has visited them has observed, many patients are kept under constant sedation. Some may need it, but most do not. Keeping patients sedated has the effect of preventing them from protesting about how they are treated. So the government is paying for drugs to prevent the government's own wards, the patients, from fighting against those who abuse them.

The operator also chooses the physicians who will be paid for attending those of his patients who do not have their own doctors. If both are unscrupulous, the result is what is known in the trade as the "gang visit": the physician whips through the nursing home in a couple of hours, glancing at only the most urgent cases, and later the government is billed as if he had given individual attention to each patient, a task requiring days, not hours. The GAO, in its Ohio investigation, found not a few examples of such gang visits. One doctor billed the government for 71 patient visits in a single day and 56 on another; he charged the taxpayers for a total of 960 patient visits in one three-month period. Another doctor billed for 487 visits to patients in a sixteen-day period, including 90 on one day and 86 on another. A podiatrist put in for 750 visits, including 32 on one Sunday. All these doctors were also handling their usual load of non-Medicaid patients. Physicians and other health professionals can also order, at government expense, goods and services that the patients clearly do not need. Of all the examples of such frauds, dug up on the all-too-rare occasions that anyone bothers to investigate, my favorite is the optometrist who tried to bill the government for an expensive pair of prescription sunglasses—for a blind patient. Others may prefer the doctor who ordered a pregnancy test—for a male patient.

The awe in which we hold the doctor makes it particularly easy for him to defraud us. Because we put him on a pedestal, and because we know he can make plenty of money legitimately, many of us think he is less likely to steal. But if Medicaid and Medicare have proved anything, it is that doctors are led into temptation just like anyone else, and that the medical profession will do what any other pressure group docs when some of its members are caught with a hand in the cookie jar—close its eyes.

The swindles we have been describing may seem petty—and taken individually they are petty—but together all those nickels and dimes add up to many millions, if not billions, of dollars a year. Nursing home operators and their collaborators can engage in these deals safely because there is little risk of being caught, and if caught, virtually no risk of being punished. Neither the GAO nor any other investigating agency has looked at more than a small fraction of the records; if the pattern found so far exists elsewhere, and there is every reason to believe it does, then there are literally millions of frauds waiting to be uncovered.

Nor are the nursing home operator and his partners punished, except in rare and extreme cases. Typically, when a government auditor catches the operator and, say, the doctor cutting a little extra on the side, all the auditor does is force them to give back the money. The case is not sent over to the district attorney for criminal prosecution, nor is any move made to lift the operator's license. The operator's explanation, usually "clerical error," is allowed to stand. This is true even when, as I have observed in a number of cases, the same operators are caught time and time again in the same types of fraud; though the explanations begin to wear thin, no attempt is made to deter the operator from trying again. There is, indeed, no reason for him not to try again. The operator knows he is not likely to get caught; that even if he is caught in one swindle he will be getting away with three others; and that in any event he runs no risk of punishment.

Beyond these types of swindles, known to those who follow the periodic Medicaid scandals, is a quite different kind of fraud, cloaked in secrecy and complexity, unknown to the public and even to many nursing home critics. Frauds at this level are the most sophisticated method of hustling the government for nursing home money. The opportunity, once perceived, has drawn into the nursing home field con men and manipulators whose skills and imagination put them in a class apart from those operators whose stealing is limited to kickbacks from pharmacies and doctors. Few of these newcomers have any experience in nursing homes or in any other aspect of the health field. All they know is how to make money, and they sense that the nursing home is a good place to exercise that talent. The identities of many are unknown, for they hide behind layers of corporate false fronts, but some of them are known, and their names, respected ones in the nursing home field, will appear in later chapters.

Their basic strategy is to manipulate the ownership and mortgaging of nursing homes receiving guaranteed government income in order to extract the most revenue and pay the least amount back in the form of income taxes. Among the costs of operating a nursing home are the costs of ownership—the amount paid out in either rent or mortgage and interest payments—costs that are reimbursed by the government when it pays for its Medicaid and Medicare patients. The higher the cost of ownership, the more the government pays. But of course the government payment does not stay with the operator; it goes on to the owner (if the operator pays rent) or to the mortgage holder (if the operator is also the owner). Thus higher ownership costs seem to benefit someone other than the operator.

Doubtless any reader with a bit of larceny in him can quickly figure out the solution. It is to make the owner appear to be someone other than the operator, while in fact the same people are collecting at both ends. If, for example, you own a nursing home, you may "sell" it to someone who turns out to be a friend or a relative of yours, then "rent" it back at a rental that requires the government to increase its payments. You split the profit between yourself as operator and yourself, in different guise, as owner. Or, alternatively, you might build a nursing home and rent it, at a very high figure, to a "nonprofit" corporation you or your friends have created. The government will pay more to that corporation, because of the high rental, than it would have paid you directly based on the cost of building the home. The extra payment comes back to you, of course, in the form of the extra high rent. Or you sell the home at an inflated price to some associates, who use the price as a basis for getting higher payments from the government. In each of these maneuvers, what you have done is find a way to increase the amount coming in by increasing the apparent cost of ownership. The same principle can be applied to other costs. You can drive up the costs of the supplies you buy by paying more than market price to suppliers that turn out to be yourself or your associates under another corporate name.

The method varies somewhat according to the way the government pays off. In a straight cost-reimbursement situation (all Medicare patients and in some states Medicaid also), the payoff is immediate, for the government pays exactly the apparent cost (plus a percentage for profit); raise the cost and the payment goes up automatically. In homes paid on flat rate so much per patient day, the payoff is not so quick. Here the nursing home industry must use the higher costs of ownership as a means of lobbying the state for an increase in the flat rate. In the almost annual bouts of lobbying over the rates, the nursing home representatives can use those costs as apparent hard evidence that they need more money. Unless the state looks behind the figures, they will appear to be convincing evidence, and since in fact the states usually just take the industry's figures and shave them a little, the contrived cost increases eventually produce the desired effect.

A universal reason for these complex transactions is to hide the incredibly high profits in the nursing home industry. For one thing, too-visible profits might undercut the poormouthing that accompanies the industry's pleas for higher rates. (Although in practice it does not seem to matter. In the late sixties, nursing homes were successfully lobbying for higher rates at the same time that stock speculators were pronouncing the industry to be the hottest thing on Wall Street.) In a broader sense, this industry, like any other, spends much of its inventive skill in trying to minimize the amount of income tax it has to pay. When you make as much money as most nursing homes do, that can be a problem. Shifts of ownership can help. If, for example, you "sell" the home at an inflated figure and then rent it back, you can take your profit as capital gains instead of regular income, and your tax will be lower. Shifting costs to the nursing home is a way of shifting profits out, into another corporation you set up for that purpose. There you may be able to diffuse the profits, perhaps by putting your family on the payroll, before the Internal Revenue can get at them. The nursing home chains, which have the best accountants, have pioneered this territory. One chain has at least five subsidiaries from which it buys goods and services.

It should be emphasized that many of these tax-avoidance ploys are legal, in contrast to the operator who does not report on his return the kickbacks he collects, Legal or not, however, it is still the taxpayer who bears the cost of the nursing homes' excessive profits.

Manipulating mortgages is another aspect of profit-making in industry and the nursing home. Despite the many protestations to the contrary, there is no safer risk than the nursing home. With guaranteed government revenue, with a growing elderly population, with a shortage of homes, there is, as the Wall Street expert said, "no way" not to make money in this business. What could be a better bet than to lend—or borrow—money against guaranteed government revenue? This is how many shoestring operators have gotten their start. If they can scrape together enough in loans (often from the original owner) for the down payment to buy a home, they can then get a first mortgage on the home at the normal interest rate of 6 to 8 percent. They know that the government revenue will carry them through and that, in fact, they can use the interest they are paying to justify higher reimbursement. If they overreach themselves, they can always cut back on service to the patients. That home can subsequently be used as collateral for second and third mortgages at much higher rates of interest. Although these interest payments can also be used as the basis for higher reimbursement, there is in fact no requirement that the money from such second and third mortgages be used for the nursing home itself.

On the contrary, the mortgage proceeds are often used for purposes that have nothing to do with taking care of sick old people. In examining the records of nursing homes in many states, I have been struck by how many profitable homes have mortgages that grow instead of decrease. Normally you would expect the home, as it makes money, to pay off its mortgage. Instead, the owners of these homes keep adding to the burden of debt that the homes are carrying. Nothing about the home indicates that the new mortgage money is spent there—on improvements, for example. Where is the money going? It is probably being used for "pyramiding," for capital for another enterprise—and there is no way of knowing what those enterprises are. In any event, guaranteed government revenue is being used for purposes foreign to patient care. From the point of view of the lender, the backing of the government provides a safe opportunity to lend money at interest far above the normal rates. Joseph Kosow of Boston, described in Chapter 6, specializes in just this kind of mortgaging.

Government revenue in effect endorses pyramiding and other dubious business practices. The sure supply of government-supported patients allows nursing home owners to take risks that other kinds of businesses could not afford. And not only that: by underwriting manipulations that artificially increase nursing home costs, the government also guarantees unnecessary increases in the rates it pays for patient care. That, too, has a double effect, for each increase in rates drives onto Medicaid people who were able to pay their own way when the rates were lower. Higher rates thus increase the number of patients supported by government as well as the rate paid for each patient. In these many ways, government policy (or lack of policy) has served to enrich nursing home owners at the expense of taxpayers and patients alike.

The link between high profits and official corruption and abuse of patients was brought out in painful detail at the hearings held by the U.S. Senate Subcommittee on Long-Term Care, held in Chicago in 1971. Most of the information came from Chicago *Tribune* reporters and investigators for a civic organization who had worked briefly in the city's nursing homes. They told of patients freezing without blankets in winter; of patients beaten at the whim of an aide; of a home that recruited its help from Chicago's derelict population; and of patients begging, amid filth and stench and degradation, for the rescue of death.

These homes were "protected" by officials who failed consistently to act against numberless violations of standards by the nursing homes. "Violations of standards" is bureaucrat language; humanity would dictate that many of those homes be razed and their owners put permanently out of business. In one home the patients were dressed in filthy rags—except on the day the inspector came. Having been duly warned of his impending arrival (a common method by which inspectors protect the operators), the management dressed the patients in good clothes, which were stored away the rest of the time. As soon as the inspector left, the good clothes went back in storage and the rags went back on the patients. An official testified that he had been made an offer (through his brother) by a nursing home owner who would pay a bounty of $100 a head for each patient sent to his nursing home.

The owners themselves testified, though reluctantly, on their profits. Benjamin Cohen was the operator who, as mentioned earlier, fed his Medicaid patients on $.78 a day. He kept them in rooms in his Kenmore Nursing Home where, according to an investigator, the stench was so great it carried as far as the dining room. But Cohen, though he protested his dedication, is not the owner as pictured by the industry's apologists: the man who sincerely wants to give patients good care, but just cannot afford it on the rate the government pays him. Under persistent questioning by Senator Charles Percy, based on information that subcommittee staff members and I had dug up in preparation for the hearing, it came out that Benjamin Cohen was doing very well indeed with his Kenmore Nursing Home. He had bought the home a few years earlier with a cash outlay of $40,000. On that investment, he had earned the previous year a net profit of $50,292—more than 100 percent in a single year. In addition, he and his wife drew salaries totaling $14,000. And there was more: the home produced for its owner a depreciation allowance (in effect, tax-free income) of $31,000. The total intake in one year, therefore, was more than twice the investment. Mr. Cohen commented: "I did not have the intention of profiteering."

Daniel A. Slader, another witness, was treasurer of the Metropolitan Chicago Nursing Home Association. He and his partners, who included his wife and another couple, owned and operated the Melbourne Nursing Home. The property was actually held in a trust agreement, which had the effect of concealing its ownership, while a separate corporation, also owned by them, operated the business. The Slader group had bought the property for $40,000 cash (Slader himself putting up $10,000 of that amount) and they were now paying themselves rent of $60,000 a year on a property worth $100,000. Senator Percy calculated that in the previous year the Slader group had made $185,248 out of the nursing home on their $40,000 investment, plus whatever depreciation advantage they enjoyed. This was a nursing home that had kept its license despite fifty recent violations and an inspector's report that found "the overall picture of the third floor to be in deplorable condition. Urine saturated beds and floor areas. The stench permeated the area . . . broken plumbing, peeling plaster, inadequate food." The last item was not surprising. In that year, while

Slader was getting rich, he was feeding his patients on $.58 a day. Senator Percy commented that Slader's business was "a good deal more profitable than any business I have seen in a long, long time." Then Percy went on to say:

> I can understand why the New York Stock Exchange is promoting nursing home stock, if this is true, but I think it is a matter of business for the Senate of the United States to determine whether this profit is an unreasonable profit and whether this profit is coming out of the hides of the old people. Whether this is coming out of their food plate. Whether this is coming out of their enjoyment of life. Whether this is coming out of just simply not painting the walls and taking care of the stench and so forth, and this is really the heart of the whole inquiry we are trying to make.

High profits and patient abuse, with government as a silent accomplice, are at the heart, also, of the inquiry I have been making for almost a decade. The operators who harvest billions in government money while neglecting their patients are the subject of profiles in the coming chapters. We shall begin with Eugene Woods, who is rare among nursing home operators: he almost got caught. Not quite, but almost.

3

Eugene Woods:
The Unsinkable Conman

EUGENE WOODS IS A LEGENDARY FIGURE in Cleveland nursing home history because of the exotic manner in which he fled the city when the roof caved in. In his business methods, Woods symbolizes the nickel-and-dime hustler. Since no one transaction is very large, this type of operator must be both inventive and energetic. He must seize every opportunity to defraud the patients and the government, letting no part of the business go unexamined for its profit potential. Thus the Woods type stands in contrast to the newer breed of nursing home profiteer, the financial manipulator who can cut himself many thousands at a single stroke. Often the perpetrators of these grand maneuvers are doing it legally, while the Woods type is required to operate on the edge of the law.

Eugene Woods once hinted at his association with organized crime. Some shady connections of his were touched upon in a memorandum of October 27, 1966, sent by the U.S. Department of Justice to the Senate Subcommittee on Long-Term Care. The memorandum stated, in part:

> The Organized Crime Division records show that in 1964 Eugene Woods was part owner in a night club in Cleveland

with one Jack Russell and Shondor Birns.* Birns has an extensive record with the Division. Mr. Mervin Gold, with whom Woods was alleged by the Cleveland *Plain Dealer* to have some connection, had frequent dealings with Birns, among them a fraudulent transaction in Canadian bonds. . . .

By the time that memorandum was written, Mervin Gold had been murdered and Eugene Woods was a refugee from the law. The senators were interested in Woods because he had owned homes in several counties in Ohio, had been indicted by a Cuyahoga County grand jury, but had evaded extradition from New Orleans to Cleveland to stand trial. The state of Ohio and Cuyahoga County officials gave up their efforts to return Eugene Woods from Louisiana in 1967. Five years later, in Baton Rouge, Woods boasted to a man he met in a bar that he had beaten a rap in a nursing home case. The stranger turned out to be a counsel for the Louisiana Health Department. He passed on the word to the proper places, where eventually the truth of Woods's boast was confirmed.

When Eugene Woods fled Ohio, he left behind him a pile of paper-filled cartons that proved to be a major archaeological find for a student of nursing home swindles. In those disorganized cartons, on scraps of paper and backs of envelopes, is the evidence of the many ways in which Woods hustled patients and governments out of their money. His methods, which I call the "Woods plan," are

---

* Jack Russell was then, and for many years, the president of the Cleveland City Council. While he held that office, he was also a partner in a business dealing in a fire protection system, widely sold to nursing home operators. Press reports said Russell was using his city position to induce businesses to buy his fire protection system. Years later, in 1972, the business appeared to have survived the risks of such exposure. The Emmanuel Care Center, a nonprofit nursing home, proposed to a foundation that it provide funding for the center to install a fire protection system purchased from the same company.

Shondor Birns (recently released from jail) has been a notorious rackets figure in the Cleveland area for many years.

practiced by many other operators all over the country, but no one else has left so extensive a record of his operations. What does not appear in the cartons was later filled in by Woods's employees and patients and those who had done business with him.

Social Security checks for his patients were a major element in the Woods plan. The amount paid a patient by Social Security is supposed to be deducted from the bill to be paid by Medicaid: if, for example, the nursing home bill is $434.00 a month, and Social Security is paying the patient $150.90 a month, Medicaid is supposed to pay the difference, $283.10 a month. The welfare caseworker is supposed to make that calculation. If the amount the patient is getting from Social Security is understated, then Medicaid can be made to pay more than it should; and if the operator handles the patient's Social Security checks, he can pocket the difference. The difference might only be $10 a month per patient, but, with one hundred patients, that adds up to $12,000 a year. It is essential, of course, that no one but the operator see the actual amount of the Social Security check.

Woods never let most of his patients even see their Social Security checks. He had his employees endorse the checks with an *X* for the patient's signature, and he cashed them himself. Later Isadore Novak, father of another nursing home operator (Sanford Novak, mentioned in Chapter 1), who had loaned Woods money, was to describe how he always tried to catch Woods on the day the Social Security and Aid for the Aged checks came in. Novak said: "I knew that he had the money on those dates and that he would pay me, because when he had the checks in his pocket and if I saw him personally I would collect, and after that he would be broke. Mr. Woods did his business from his pocket, and if you were there when he received his patients' checks, he would just endorse the checks over to his creditors." At one point Woods reduced his chances of being caught by arranging to have some of his patients' checks made out to an organization, Senior Citizens Club of America, of which he was head. These included retroactive checks totaling thousands of dollars.

The Woods plan covered more than Social Security. Once he billed the estate of a deceased patient for $7,000 for care at a rate that had been "orally" determined between Woods and the patient: there was no record for the administrator of the estate to check. Like so many other operators, he filched the personal funds of his patients: a note reading "Received of petty cash $100, charge to Schwartz account" is a reminder that one Schwartz had just been billed $100 for Woods's pocket money. Someone was even indentured to Woods, as shown in this note: "I will stay and work for Mr. Woods for room, board, clothes and cigarettes." In some papers Woods appears as a prospector noting veins of gold for future development. There was, for example, a listing of all the coins in a collection belonging to one of his patients, asterisks pinpointing the most valuable items. Another paper listed the insurance policies held by residents, noting the value of each and the names of the insurers.

Woods's cartons contained the raw material for a dozen indictments, but the county prosecutor chose to follow up only one case of defrauding a patient. When Woods was indicted on that charge, it seemed to spell the end of an operation that at various times included ten nursing homes, a drugstore, and several other businesses.

Operating nursing homes was a Woods family tradition. In 1940 his father and his mother, a nurse, entered the business with their Norrwood Christian Home in Norwalk, Ohio. Eugene himself ran that home for a time, with the assistance of a petite young blond nurse named Angela Mahl, later to figure significantly in his life. At Norrwood, Woods was charged with various violations of licensure regulations, ranging from failing to comply with orders to protect his patients from fire hazards to neglecting to obtain a food license. These uncorrected violations did not, however, prompt authorities to shut down the nursing home.

From his Norrwood home, Eugene Woods moved out to new enterprises. He bought an old toy factory in New London, Ohio, and converted it into a nursing home, which he called the Norrwood Hospital, a title that was illegal as well as inaccurate. Education was one of the attractions of the institution—a so-called "complete course" in practical nursing. Uninhibited by a state law requiring the accreditation of schools offering practical nurse training, Woods's unaccredited school turned out "graduates," giving each an impressive pin-and-diploma set of original design.

His "hospital" established, Woods next launched his operations in Cleveland with the opening of a retirement home at the St. Regis Hotel there. Newspaper articles reported on the air of bustling activity at the old, seven-story hotel on Cleveland's upper Euclid Avenue, a red brick arsenal of a building in the heart of the prostitution district. The nursing home operator loved to regale visitors to his home with colorful accounts of life in his retirement facility. His program of activities even included the wedding of two elderly residents who had met, fallen in love, and courted beneath the roof of the St. Regis.

A business associate of Woods in the St. Regis enterprise was a man who today is still operating nursing homes in Cleveland and southern Ohio. He is Sidney Garfield, who has served as the vice-president of the Northeast Ohio Nursing Home Association. One of his homes in Troy, Ohio, was purchased from Eugene Woods; the quality of service he renders has occasioned bitter complaints from families and patients. Woods's connections with other operators were not limited to his alliance with Garfield. Joined in a partnership with Alvin Klein and Milton Wolfson, the owners of six nursing homes, Eugene Woods was co-incorporator with them of the Hotel Howe in Akron. This run-down hostelry had been converted into a home for the elderly but extended its hospitality to others, urging truck drivers, for instance, to stop there for a night's rest. In time the Akron Health Department showed some concern about the situation, charging that the shabby hotel was actually being illegally operated as a nursing home. Garfield, Klein, and Wolfson continue in the nursing home business today; indeed, in 1972 Wolfson and a group that included the past president of the "Young Presidents of America" bought a dozen nursing homes in Florida.

Among Woods's allegedly nonprofit enterprises was a home called the Weddell House. The goals of that establishment were set forth grandiloquently in its Articles of Incorporation with this statement of purpose: "Aid in Religious and monetary help to those in need of it and to provide lodging, food, and care and all things necessary and incidental thereto." Besides "all things necessary," its lodgers were offered the inspiration of having on the premises a cumbersome, ornate bed, in which Abraham Lincoln supposedly slept one night.

Eugene Woods's operations continued to grow and multiply. Across the city from the St. Regis Hotel, he leased an automobile repair garage, which he transformed into a nursing home and named the Charles Woods Memorial Hospital. In later years, under the new management of Max Strauss and with a new name, the Riverside Nursing Home, that institution was the subject of another Cleveland newspaper exposé. (Max Strauss is the subject of the next chapter.)

Next, Eugene Woods leased a place called the Regent Hotel from a corporation of which he himself was an officer. (One of the principals of that corporation, Percy D. Harvey, was later indicted on charges of fraud in connection with a Small Business Administration loan.)

At the Regent Hotel, Woods and his brother, the Reverend Hilton Woods, opened what they named the Senior

Citizens Club of America, where, the club newspaper reported, the Reverend Hilton served as both chaplain and decorator, and Miss Angela Mahl, the blond nurse from the Norrwood Christian Home, served as assistant administrator.

The good life enjoyed by residents of the Regent was reflected in the columns of the house organ, *The Golden Times,* which faithfully reported on the doings of Eugene Woods. For example, the second issue of the paper had this to say of him:

> Eugene Woods possesses a special skill in making friends and influencing senior citizens. He spices his personal and business contacts with "horse sense," perhaps better, "Woods sense" and a pungent wit. The combination gets results. . . .
>
> Recreation and religious but nonsectarian programs of many kinds appear, so to speak, at the drop of the Administrator's sometimes unique hats. He is especially fond of a high crowned Hawaiian cap with vizor made of red and yellow straw. . . . Cheerily and with apparent casualness, wanted projects—a gift shop, a game room, even this newspaper—become realities. And in the midst of seeming confusion, the Administrator will sit down at the beautiful organ in Castle Lounge, the new dining room, and play old hymns so movingly that residents on other floors, hearing the music, assemble for a "sing fest." Many will assure you that they "just love Mr. Woods."

They just loved Mr. Woods, though Mr. Woods was robbing them in ways that were not particularly subtle. Elderly people, especially in nursing homes, are easy victims of conmen like Woods and so many other nursing home operators. Some are senile, and all have lost contact with the world outside. So, while his hand was in their pockets, the members of the Senior Citizens Club of America continued to lavish their praise on Woods, in their house organ and sometimes in the daily papers. Occasionally the papers published pictures of Woods and his elderly flock. One such picture showed the group, including Woods and other nursing home operators, floating down the Cuyahoga River on a river boat called *The Goodtime.*

The times appeared very good indeed for the founder of the Senior Citizens Club, at whose residence gaiety flourished in the religious aura created by the live-in decorator-chaplain, the Reverend Hilton Woods. Eugene Woods's domain spread beyond nursing homes. He operated Weddell House, a residence hotel from which welfare recipients were shuffled in and out of his nursing homes. He was the owner of the Players' Theatre, a night club-theatre whose patrons were entertained by performers as they dined. With Angela Mahl as business partner, he entered into negotiations, under the name of Eugene Mahl, to purchase an old Cleveland estate to be converted into his eleventh nursing home operation. He also owned a sagging frame nursing home called the Sunnyside, which he leased to a dentist, and in a large downtown department store he operated a concession offering Amish foods for sale. Credit seemed universally available to him.

That was Eugene Woods's successful position when the office of Aid for the Aged in Cleveland received an anonymous telephone call. The caller reported that a patient in need of medical attention was being housed at the Regent—illegally so, since the hotel was licensed only as a residence, not as a nursing home. A caseworker from Aid for the Aged rode out to the Regent, and the drama opened.

The public knew nothing of the incident for a week. Then the Cleveland *Plain Dealer* published the first of countless installments of the story. The newspaper reported that the caseworker, searching for the sick resident, had to break down the door of her bedroom. She found the old woman huddled behind a barricade made of a bureau and bed; she was senile, and her hands were bleeding where she had dug her nails into her palms. The next day the caseworker returned, this time accompanied by a group of her fellow workers, to see if others were being held at the hotel illicitly. Eugene Woods met the group at the door and refused to let them into the residents' quarters. When the caseworkers called the sheriff, Woods had to let them in, but he fought a delaying action by blocking the elevators and misdirecting them in the halls. The caseworkers, their work unfinished, left, saying they would be back on Monday to complete the investigation.

That was on Friday. On Sunday, the day before the caseworkers were due to return, Woods packed up about thirty Regent residents and moved them out of Cleveland, to his Hotel Howe in Akron. It was a strange action, for Woods had not informed the relatives of the people he moved, nor had he informed the caseworkers who had assigned them to the Regent, although—or perhaps because—he was moving the people out of the caseworkers' jurisdiction. The ones he did not take were in effect abandoned. The Red Cross was called in to take care of the ones he left behind, until their records were untangled and they were assigned to nursing homes.

The astonishing story of how those elderly men and women had been transported to that old hotel, thirty miles away, stirred up several official theories for Woods's conduct. The chief probate judge suggested that Woods would be found to have misused funds under a number of legal guardianships he held for some of his residents; this was later confirmed. An assistant county prosecutor reasoned that Woods skipped town because of his many debts; later it came out that he did indeed owe money all around town. The chief attorney for the Veterans Administration said he suspected some members of the underworld and other nursing home operators shared a desire to see Woods out of town, so that he could not be brought to trial and forced to testify about connections between the nursing home industry and organized crime. But no single explanation was ever decided upon, and no one knew why Woods had so carelessly left those damning cartons of records behind. One theory was that he might have left them to divert attention from still more damning records that he might have taken with him.

In Akron, a few days after Woods's arrival, one of his patients was found wandering in the streets and was traced to Cleveland. This led to a charge against Woods of operating the Hotel Howe as a nursing home without a license. When the police arrived at the Hotel Howe with a warrant for Woods's arrest, they found the place padlocked and Woods gone. He had taken off again, about a week after he had left Cleveland. This time he had taken fifteen of his thirty charges and moved them another fifty miles, to the Ashland Terrace Motor Hotel in Ashland, Ohio. This hotel was owned by one Adolph Tuckey, who, according to the chief legal counsel for the Ohio Department of Health, had some business connections with Woods. Somehow word reached the health department of Woods's new location, but apparently word also reached Woods that the health department was sending a team to the motel. One hour before their arrival he vanished, taking with him only Miss Angela Mahl, his twenty-nine-year-old nurse. Back in Cuyahoga County, the prosecutor announced that Woods could be fined $25 for every day he had operated the Hotel Regent as an unlicensed nursing home, and declared he was considering filing such a charge against Woods. That charge was never filed. In the office of the Cuyahoga County recorder, it was discovered that Woods owed the United States more than $21,000 in federal taxes and that there were nine liens against his Senior Citizens Club. Employees at the Regent complained that their wages had not been paid. And almost daily, fresh rumors were heard that Woods had been spotted in various places.

In the Regent Hotel, a locked room yielded the boxes of papers left behind by Woods. Among those papers was discovered the crucial evidence on which the Veterans Administration built a criminal case against Eugene Woods for bilking a veteran.

The patient was John Huggins, a World War I veteran, housed at the Norrwood Christian Home in Norwalk. Woods had filed papers, notarized by Angela Mahl, giving him power of attorney over Huggins's affairs. Armed with this authority, he withdrew Huggins's savings of $15,000 from a Canton, Ohio, bank, and sold the veteran's stock in the Home Savings and Loan Company in Canton, valued at about $14,000. Thus it appeared that Woods had taken the old man for close to $30,000. It did not seem likely that Huggins had willingly put himself at Woods's mercy. According to the assistant county prosecutor, Woods and his brother had plucked the old veteran out of a roominghouse and driven him to their nursing home, threatening to turn him over to the authorities on a charge of falsifying a claim for relief when he was receiving a veteran's pension. Hug-gins, like many older people who become the victims of nursing home operators, was an easy mark. Mildly confused, he was doubtless frightened by the assertion that he had violated a law he did not fully understand, and he was not strong enough to resist when, on a wintry day, they took off his shoes (as reported by the janitor of the building where Huggins lived, who noted the license plate when he saw the Woods brothers taking the old man away). As to how Woods lighted upon Huggins as a profitable victim, a VA official suspected that someone at the local Soldiers and Sailors Relief Agency had tipped Woods off that there was a target with money available. The VA official also reported a rumor that Woods had used truth serum to get Huggins to tell him where his money was. (John Huggins did not live to see the outcome of the case against Eugene Woods. He died only a few months after Woods left town.)

On the basis of evidence produced by the Veterans Administration, the county grand jury in Cleveland indicted Woods in absentia on charges of larceny by trick for having appropriated the savings of Mr. Huggins. Then the Veterans Administration official who was working to build up more evidence in the case told me he had been called off by Washington. This irate official told me his investigation had produced information that Woods had grossed $1 million in a single year and that he owned a yacht. Then he indignantly added that Woods conveyed food in open garbage pails in unrefrigerated vehicles between his homes in Cleveland and Norwalk, eighty miles away.

The indictment was issued, but no one seemed able to find Eugene Woods. The Veterans Administration investigation stopped. The case ground to a halt.

Though Woods himself was not available, the evidence against the missing man continued to pile up. By searching through the records, including Woods's famous cartons, and by hearing the accounts of his victims who came forward after he had fled, I learned the infinite variety of hustles practiced by Woods during his Cleveland career. Most notable among these was the method Woods used to silence any troublesome patients or employees. His strategy was to discount any complaint as coming from someone who was mentally unbalanced. At one level, that simply means telling anyone responding to such a complaint something like, "Oh, he's just senile," but Woods used a more sinister method to blot out what they had to say. He was prone to having his critics "probated"—that is, declared mentally incompetent in court. Old people of course are sometimes senile, more often mildly confused; that does not mean they are not valid witnesses to the personal abuse they have suffered. But if the operator can, with the help of cooperative caseworkers and physicians, get them committed to a mental institution, then no testimony they give against him will be believed by courts or investigators. This method was to crop up again and again as I studied the nursing home industry. When I raised the subject with a California investigator, he said:

"Hell, they even do it to free a bed for a patient who can pay more."

Anna Schroeder was a classic example of this technique. She was an unhappy resident at the Woods-operated St. Regis Hotel, who complained to the police that Woods had appropriated her money. The police responded with a perfunctory investigation and reported in their record:

> At Room 430 talked to Anna. Anna is hard of hearing and had a speech defect. Anna said she lived in Amherst, Ohio, until 4 years ago when she fell down and fractured her hip. She was taken to Norrwood Christian Home [operated by Woods] to be treated and recuperate. She had $10,000 in the bank at that time. Since then her money had been dwindling. She admitted spending some of it to live on. She said she turned the remainder of her account over to the owner-operator, Eugene Woods.

While the police investigator was laboring to get Mrs. Schroeder's story, made difficult by her physical handicaps, the persuasive Woods burst into Mrs. Schroeder's room. Once in the room, Woods calmly explained his use of her money. She cursed him in a shrill voice for taking her money; one can almost hear the contrast of Woods's even-paced voice as he continued to recount the disposal of the funds. Her care, he said, cost about $1,800 a year. Ultimately her bank account did not cover her expenses; with gallantry he had written off a part of her costs as a bad debt. He had the gall to add that he had relieved her grateful family of their responsibility by taking her, a difficult, disagreeable person, into his nursing home.

The policeman asked for the records of her expenses. His confidence in Woods was apparently not shaken by his not having them available; he would, he promised, assemble the records the next week.

On the policeman's second visit, Woods gave him a

copy of a financial statement. It was computed on the invoice stationery of another Woods-operated home, the Norrwood Hospital, in another city—New London, Ohio—in which Mrs. Schroeder had never been a patient, a detail that passed unnoticed by the police. The invoice indicated that, on the day following her admission, Woods drew from her account, on a cashier's check, almost $4,000. The bill continued, itemizing monthly payments for nursing home care over a period of two and a half years and ending with the last three months of care unpaid. She was charged, on this statement, for medications at the rate of $100 a month for the first four months. Then all charges for medications stopped.

Not until six months after she entered the nursing home was she visited by a physician. When the doctor finally did see her, he found her to be suffering from hypertension and to be mentally deficient. She remained a nursing home patient for another two years. Then, when her savings were all gone, she was miraculously found to be cured and able to live on welfare payments in a Woods-managed hotel, the St. Regis.

None of this sequence struck the police as being unusual. The investigator never questioned Woods's right to an immediate withdrawal of $4,000 on the presumption that Mrs. Schroeder would need that amount of care in the future. The investigator never saw that the presumption was made by Woods—that neither a physician's diagnosis nor recommendation for such care accompanied the withdrawal of the money.

On the policeman's second visit, Woods resorted to a trick commonly used by nursing home operators: a recantation by the patient. Woods showed a statement, neatly typed, saying, "This is to acknowledge that I understand the disbursement of my funds and that my bank account is closed. The funds have been used to provide for my care."

Signed "Mrs. Anna M. Schroeder." That ended it. The police investigation was closed with the terse statement: "Warned Anna."

The police never asked themselves if "Anna," as they always referred to her, had any choice other than signing the statement for "Mr. Woods," as the police always referred to him. If for no other reasons than that she had no more money, she had no choice.

Mrs. Schroeder complained, again, to the police. She wrote that she did not see her Social Security checks and "they never let me sign it—they do it downstairs." She added that ominous note, a constant theme of both patients and their relatives, "Don't tell I wrote you. Please help." The police again responded. In response to their second inquiry, Woods fell back on the last bastion of nursing home operators. He would, he said, probably probate Mrs. Schroeder. "She is getting so troublesome," he rationalized. Mrs. Anna Schroeder never complained again.

Mary Burrows was an employee who complained and was silenced. A black woman in her late thirties, she had lost her job as a stenographer in the 1958 recession. She went for help to the county welfare department, which, instead of the usual action of referring her to the state employment office, sent her to Woods's St. Regis Nursing Home, where she was hired and sent across the street to a vacant house Woods used as his office.

On her third day at work, Mrs. Burrows's troubles began with a seemingly petty incident. Eugene Woods presented her with some checks made out to patients in his nursing home, instructing her to endorse the checks with an X, and to witness that endorsement as if the check had been so endorsed by the patients.

Mary Burrows was upset, convinced that to do as she was asked would be not only illegal but immoral and contrary to divine law. Fearfully, she endorsed the checks, but disturbed by the impropriety of her action, she wrote Ohio's governor, Michael DiSalle. Later, she gave me a copy of his reply, which said, in part: ". . . In further reference to your letter, we have received information that the method of handling checks at the St. Regis is not an authorized procedure. The Cuyahoga County Aid for the Aged office has been informed of the situation and the problem is being studied. . . ."

Meanwhile, Mrs. Burrows called the county welfare department, saying she would not return to that job. She recounted that, in the vacant house where Woods put her to work, she saw signs of human presence in the form of unmade beds on the second floor, but she never saw the people who evidently lived there. She said she had seen no less than three guns on the premises, plus boxes she believed to contain narcotics,

Owed three days' pay by Woods, but afraid to go alone to collect it, she asked the police to accompany her. As they were leaving the office with her, the police commented on Woods's questionable activities, saying he actually belonged in prison.

Shortly thereafter, Mary Burrows lost her freedom. Two policemen arrived at her apartment, without prior warning, and drove her to the state mental hospital in Cleveland. Within a few days she was taken to the probate court, where, after a hearing lasting approximately fifteen minutes, she was committed to the mental institution. She had had no legal counsel; the only physician to examine her had been a court physician who had asked her a few questions. She was hospitalized for what she was told was further treatment of a mental illness—an illness about which she had never before been informed.

The case for Mary Burrows's commitment was presented by a caseworker from the county welfare department, to which she had gone so recently for help. A city doctor, whom she at no time saw, scrawled a note on a prescription form for the welfare department, suggesting that she suffered from severe psychoneurosis and possibly early schizophrenia. That doctor recommended probate action. His report on the unseen patient opened the action against Mary Burrows, but the medical report by the court physician was quite as damaging, even though it embraced contradictions and factual errors. On the form he was required to complete on Mrs. Burrows, he declared her speech to be distinct and coherent, her motor activity normal. She was not, he noted, overactive, depressed, or irritable. But she was suspicious, he said, although he failed to fill in the space on that form asking for indications of illusions or suspicions. Instead, he jotted down the inscrutable notation, "The Negro race is jealous and envious of me." Then, after stating that the patient was "normal," he added: "Excitable, cries easily, can't hold down job, thinks everyone against her, persecution complex, depressed and obsessed with sex." (Apparently the word had not reached him that Mrs. Burrows had worked for some time as a secretary in a steel company.) He then went on to state that Mrs. Burrows claimed the welfare department had sent her to work in a vacant house where there were three guns (which was true). The police had had to accompany her to get her pay. She believed the place had something to do with narcotics. The report closed with a recommendation of hospitalization because of "flight of ideas—confused."

In her report, the county caseworker listed Mrs. Burrows's last job as having been with the steel company, neglecting altogether to mention the job with Eugene Woods to which the county office had assigned her. She stated her opinion that Mrs. Burrows's illness seemed to result from her being black, called her emotional, reported she cried constantly, claimed she might become violent, stated that someone had said her mother had been confined to a mental institution (a confinement for which no record can be found), and added that Mrs. Burrows had admitted to having been a prostitute.

On such claims and charges, unattended by either a lawyer or her own doctor, judged by individuals who did not know her, Mrs. Burrows was hospitalized for a ninety-day probation period. Ohio law provides that if a patient is treated and released within that period, there is no permanent record of probation. For Mrs. Burrows, things were different. Just before the ninety-day period expired, the hospital submitted to the court a report stating that, according to the hospital's evaluation, she was oriented and not intellectually impaired. But the director of the hospital wrote in a letter: "She did show strong and bizarre ideas of a grandiose and persecutory nature." Because, he said, she suffered from a psychosis of the paranoid schizophrenic type, the director recommended that she be declared insane and committed to institutional care. So Mary Burrows was permanently probated.

One month later, however, her insanity now permanently on the records, she was suddenly released from that same institution. The same court physician who had filled out the commitment form now found her miraculously cured. The same court declared her to be competent.

But no one could undo the damage to Mary Burrows— and the fact that Woods was now protected from her testimony. The diagnosis of insanity was permanently on her record. Hence, in any future inquiry into Eugene Woods's activities, her testimony would be inadmissible. Her record will follow her all her life, available to potential employers. (After her release, Mrs. Burrows passed a Civil Service examination for a clerical position, but has never been hired.)

It seems clear that the county welfare agency that assigned patients to Woods's nursing homes, that overlooked his habit of illegally signing patients' checks, and that had

sent Mary Burrows to him as an employee, was also directly responsible for her commitment after she informed on
Woods to the governor.

TWO YEARS LATER, the FBI discovered Woods in Baton
Rouge, Louisiana. He was going by the name of Eugene
Frederick, living in a trailer with Angela Mahl, wearing a
moustache disguise, running a restaurant, and "planning
to open a rest home." Placed under $25,000 bond (quickly
reduced to $7,500), Woods said he would welcome extra-
dition to Ohio.

The rest is a mystery. Ohio's governor, James Rhodes, signed invalid extradition papers for him and sent
them to Louisiana's governor, John J. McKeithen. After
many statements and puzzling maneuvers, Woods was finally set free by a New Orleans district judge, Edward A.
Haggerty, Jr. Ohio had tried (presumably) and lost, on the
technicality that the state failed to notarize its request for
extradition.

In an interview in New Orleans before the final hearing
on his extradition, Woods expatiated on several subjects. He
chastised social workers, defended his own attitudes toward
the elderly, and may have helped explain some of His own
success by bragging to reporters: "Carlos Marcello [a reputed top Mafia figure in Louisiana] and Shondor Birns [the
Cleveland rackets figure] keep things under control."

That Woods might thereby have explained the forces
behind his ultimate freedom from the law is indicated in a
memorandum issued by a staff member of the Senate Special Committee on Aging:

Among the attorneys representing Eugene Woods in his effort to block his extradition from Louisiana were John F.
Rau, Jr., and G. Wray Gill, Sr.

G. Wray Gill . . . is also Carlos Marcello's principal

attorney. This information was given to Wendell Lindsey (Senator Long's office) by the Assistant District Attorney in Orleans Parish. He also stated that the District Attorney in Jefferson Parish was primarily responsible for arguing the extradition case, had made a very half-hearted effort, and did not seem to be really interested in the case against Woods.

The Assistant District Attorney in Orleans Parish also said there were rumors about to the effect that a large sum of money had been offered to prevent Woods' extradition. He did not say by whom or to whom the offer was allegedly made.

Woods was free, but Governor Rhodes of Ohio told reporters that the case was not closed, that the state would renew its effort to bring Woods back for trial. Nothing of the sort happened. Five years later, in 1971, I asked the assistant Cuyahoga County prosecutor, Dennis McGuire, about the status of the case. His response was: "If you can find him, it's active." It was a strange position for the prosecution to take. It did not seem to me that it would be hard for the Ohio authorities to find Woods; he had been doing business openly in Louisiana, and there was no reason to think he had gone underground after the failure of the attempt to extradite him. On the other hand, it did not seem likely that I, an individual, would ever find him. Yet that in a sense is what happened.

Eugene Woods bobbed to the surface again in January 1972. Still in Louisiana, he had declared his intention to apply for a license to get back into the nursing home business. I learned about Woods's reappearance from an HEW official in Washington. The administrator of nursing home licensing and certification in Louisiana had called HEW to check upon one Eugene Woods who planned to apply for permission to operate a nursing home in Baton Rouge. A vague recollection attaching to that name had led the administrator to check with HEW, whose representative in turn asked me to call the Louisiana official on the chance that I might be able to assist in the identification of the applicant. So opened the last chapter in the story of Eugene Woods, and the last was not unlike the first.

I called the Louisiana official, Jack Letcher, who held the title of Administrator, Licensing and Certification Division, in Louisiana's State Department of Hospitals at Baton Rouge. His story went thus: A man named Eugene Woods, the operator of the Fisherman's Wharf restaurant in Baton Rouge, had discussed with a director of the Louisiana Health Department the feasibility of applying for a license to operate a nursing home in a building that was being converted from a funeral home. Then, in a barroom conversation, Woods told a stranger who turned out to be a health department lawyer that he'd been in some trouble with nursing homes elsewhere, but had "beaten the rap" and was ready to get back into the business. The attorney passed on this information to Letcher, who vaguely recalled how, some years before, his office had been contacted by the Subcommittee on Long-Term Care, seeking information on the whereabouts of the fugitive Woods. Letcher called HEW and they called me.

I outlined to Mr. Letcher the highlights of Eugene Woods's escapades and his final victory over the threat of his extradition to Ohio, whereupon we agreed that I would send a picture of Woods, along with whatever other identifying information I could assemble. I obtained copies of two pictures the Cleveland *Press* had published, and sent these to Letcher along with a copy of Woods's signature and several news stories out of the many that had appeared. One article told how a Louisiana sheriff had identified Woods through his having a partially amputated thumb; another was the report on the operator's remark about Carlos Marcello. (Letcher had told me that Marcello himself had once run an unlicensed nursing home in Louisiana that authorities were unable to close, despite numerous attempts.)

Very shortly, I heard from Letcher the news I had anticipated. He wrote, in a letter dated January 31,1972:

> The picture was the evidence that assured us that the person
> represented in the articles is the same one that contacted us
> relative to conversion of a building to be used as a nursing
> home.
>   . . . We are concerned that he has only been charged
> but never convicted. Since you are interested and since
> Ohio has a vested interest in the case, we will keep you
> informed. . . .

In Mr. Letcher's letter, I thought I had found the confir-
mation needed to renew Ohio's action against the man who
had flouted its laws.

Impelled by the declaration of Cuyahoga County's assistant prosecutor, Dennis McGuire, that if I could find Eugene
Woods, the case against him was "active," I then called the
county prosecutor's office. Mr. McGuire was ill, but very shortly the chief prosecutor, John T. Corrigan, returned my call.

The prosecutor spent some time telling me how Louisiana draws its law from Spanish or Roman sources, as distin-
guished from English sources—an explanation he seemed
to offer for Cuyahoga County's failure to extradite Eugene
Woods from Louisiana. Two of the county's police officers
had twice gone to Louisiana, be reported, but he described
their fate in the same metaphor he was later to use to a reporter: "We got the fast shuffle."

Prosecutor Corrigan (who had also been the county
prosecutor at the time of Woods's indictment by the grand
jury) seemed determined to disallow that the county had
had a case, even at the beginning. In a later conversation,
Dennis McGuire, the assistant prosecutor, expressed equally
little optimism about bringing Eugene Woods back to face
the charges against him. The heart of the difficulty was that
John Huggins was dead, for as McGuire said, "Without the

old man's testimony, we couldn't get anyplace." What was overlooked by McGuire was the fact that if there was now no case because the veteran was dead, then none existed in 1966, during the abortive extradition proceedings. Huggins had then been dead for two years.

In retrospect, one can scarcely avoid the conclusion that the prosecutor's office had not actually wanted to bring Eugene Woods to trial. Nor were Louisiana officials, pitted against Carlos Marcello's lawyers, any more energetic in their pursuit of justice. With such half-hearted opposition, crowned by a technical error in the Ohio governor's bid for extradition, Eugene Woods was free.

There the situation rests, as of this writing. Not much has changed. The government officials appear to be frozen in the same paralysis that immobilized them five years ago. Eugene Woods, still creative enough to see the potential for turning a mortuary into a nursing home, has accomplished his boast to the Louisiana lawyer. Assisted by official indifference, he has indeed "beaten the rap."

Scanty reports from Louisiana indicate that, as of early 1973, Woods was about halfway back into the nursing home business. He had not yet applied for a license, but he had been involved in an abortive deal to buy a home in New Orleans, the Ruth Ellen Nursing Home, owned by Mrs. Ruth Begnaud. According to Mrs. Begnaud, Woods worked for her as "food supervisor" for a couple of months late in 1972, and Woods's friend Angela Mahl worked for her as a nurse. Mrs. Begnaud complained that Woods would order equipment at her expense and have it delivered to a boarding-house he was supposedly buying. They parted company without consummating the agreement under which Woods was going to buy Mrs. Begnaud's home. As he left, she said, Woods took three of her patients away to his boarding-house. Mrs. Begnaud told me she had wanted to take Woods to court, but that her lawyer advised her she would lose, because Woods was represented by John F. Rau, Jr., who had earlier represented Woods along with an attorney for the reputed Mafioso Carlos Marcello. It did not seem that moving south had changed Eugene Woods's ways of doing business.

Not much had changed in Woods's old territory, either, Indeed, four years after he left town, an event reminiscent of his days took place in one of his old nursing homes, the St. Regis. Renamed the Midtown Nursing Home, it was home to, among others, the Reverend Robert Walker, a retired black minister in his eighties.

The penniless Reverend Walker, diagnosed as confused and sent to Midtown for his protection, was so ineffectively supervised that, unnoticed, he opened a door from his floor onto an outside fire escape, seven floors above the ground. Then, it was theorized, he climbed up an unguarded open steel ladder to the eighth floor and entered, through an unlocked door, into an attic area, from which, perhaps seeking warmth, he crawled through a ten-inch opening into a small space. There he lay, and there he died, shriveling to a skeleton, undetected for thirteen months.

After the body was accidentally discovered by a workman, public attention centered on the mystery of how Walker's absence from the home, and the body's presence in the attic, had gone so long unnoticed. Given the drama of the case, no one was excited about its humdrum financial details. Yet those details are of particular interest to the student of nursing home frauds.

For eight months after Reverend Walker disappeared, the home did not report his absence to the state and continued to collect its monthly payments for the support of the missing man. The reason they stopped collecting after eight months was that a caseworker, making a routine count of her patients, discovered that Reverend Walker was no longer there. Each month, also, a separate state check for $11 made out to Walker himself, was sent to the home: $8 for his personal expense money, $3 for his Medicare coverage (although in fact he never was covered by Medicare). The home also failed to return those checks for the full thirteen months from the time Walker disappeared to when his body was discovered.

In time the state deducted from Midtown's payments the amount due for the eight extra months of support that the home had collected, a total of $1,897.50. That was all the state did. It did not impose a penalty of any kind; it did not even collect interest on its money. As for those $11 monthly checks, the state did not even try to get that money back. Not only did the nursing home evade any punishment for collecting for a nonexistent patient; it actually came out ahead.

Thus, for the old Eugene Woods nursing home and for the state alike, business went on as usual.

4

Max Strauss:
The Nickel and Dimer

A RELATIVELY SMALL NURSING HOME, tucked away inconspicuously in a drab Cleveland neighborhood, once briefly served to instruct the community in some major facts about the business. Riverside Nursing Home, operated at one time by the departed Eugene Woods, rose from obscurity to become the subject of a front-page expose in the Cleveland *Press.* The expose led, in time, to investigations by the state and federal governments, a federal grand jury investigation, and pompous official pronouncements, and ended with the operator remaining in business, still licensed.

Riverside Nursing Home had been built as an automobile repair garage—a boxlike structure with a gas station as its neighbor. Eugene Woods leased it for its potential as a nursing home, blocked out small bedrooms, installed a few small bathrooms, and opened for business. He named the operation the Charles Woods Memorial Hospital, and after he moved on to other enterprises, a new operator arrived on the scene—Max Strauss.

Like many other operators, Strauss entered the nursing home field from an inconspicuous and unprofitable business, in his case leather manufacturing. When that operation failed, he moved into his nursing home career, where he would enjoy the assurance of government support to ward off a repetition of his recent failure. His new business showed troubling portents. Inspectors regularly notified him of violations in his operation, to no avail—for, unruffled, Strauss was financially able, one year after he leased Riverside, to plan an expansion of his business. Then, one summer day in 1968, a telephone call launched Max Strauss toward unwelcome prominence.

Riverside, for me, was the place where I added greatly to the knowledge of nursing home swindles that I had dug out of the cartons left behind by Eugene Woods when he fled town. I was to find that Max Strauss had made imaginative variations on the basic Woods plan for extracting extra money from the government—which were not all original with Strauss, however, for I was to find them practiced all over the country. Most important, I got through Riverside a glimpse into the possible national magnitude of the nursing home hustle. With the help of a cooperative official, I was able to go through an entire month's Medicaid transactions at Riverside—which involved reading some fifty pages of computer printouts and comparing the payments recorded there with the known status of Riverside patients. I was able to calculate that Max Strauss had collected an extra 23 percent from various sources in that month. That figure is probably incomplete, for it did not include any possible swindles that would not show up on the Medicaid records, nor does it include what the government loses on those patients at Riverside who do not need to be there—the healthy patient racket.

For one small nursing home, the amount involved is not impressive. Strauss got an extra $1,061.70 that month, beyond his government revenue of $7,000 a month. The annual amount of $12,000, if that was a typical month, seems small compared to the other misuses of public money that go on in this country. But suppose that figure is typical of nursing homes in general—and everything I have seen in the last few years leads me to believe it *is* typical—then the amount involved becomes frighteningly large. The nursing home industry has an income of $3.5 billion (as of 1972). If we apply to that amount the figure of 23 percent padding, we have to conclude that taxpayers and relatives of nursing home patients are losing $800 million a year to the operators in thousands of nickel-and-dime swindles. And that is a lot of money.

Max Strauss had many stratagems to increase his income at government expense. One was practiced on patients who came to Riverside with some money of their own, often a lump-sum payment from Social Security or the Veterans Administration, Strauss would open a bank account for such a patient, the account being controlled by the operator rather than the patient. Strauss would then pay himself for the patient's care at a rate higher than Medicaid, and when the account had been emptied he would put the patient on Medicaid. Strauss also found ways to exceed the legal twenty-eight-bed capacity of his home. He had a folding bed in which he kept one extra patient, and another patient, listed as living at Riverside, was actually being kept in her home by a nurse employed by Strauss. And on at least one occasion, Strauss collected from Medicaid for a patient who was being supported in a hospital by Medicare. Like Eugene Woods, Max Strauss intercepted his patients' Social Security checks. Although Strauss did not have Woods's political connections, he took the precaution of making personal loans to the caseworker who covered his nursing home, and he had no trouble with that office. But none of these practices at the Riverside home came to light until I had been through a long investigation that began—like the exposure of Eugene Woods—with an anonymous telephone call.

The caller informed reporter Paul Lilley of the Cleveland *Press* that Max Strauss was pursuing some highly irregular practices at Riverside Nursing Home. He was, the caller said, mishandling Social Security and welfare checks and making interest-free loans to himself from twenty-three of his patients' private bank accounts.*

Paul Lilley discussed these allegations with members of the county welfare department and was told that what he had heard was probably nonsense. However, the department offered its services in checking out the story. Lilley invited me to accompany them on a visit to Riverside. Thus, four of us—a member of the legal department of county welfare, its public relations officer, Paul Lilley, and I—went to call on Max Strauss.

We found him to be a soft-spoken, middle-aged man, not at all affecting the bombastic speech of some of his peers in the business. The county employees, verging persistently on apology, asked Strauss a few simple questions concerning his operation of Riverside. At the end they thanked him for his cooperation, and after we had departed, they lectured the reporter for having wasted their time in pursuit of a patently insubstantial rumor. One of them said to Lilley, "You certainly have nothing here. We wish every home was operated as well as this, and financial records were kept as well as his."

But Lilley and I were left with nagging doubts about what we had observed in our flying review of Max Strauss's records. Convinced we had spotted discrepancies in the patients' records, we agreed to make a return visit, and unattended by the welfare personnel, we went back to ask Max Strauss some additional questions.

At first he allowed us to look through the folders he kept on each of his patients. We were able to discover five

* Under Ohio law, welfare patients are permitted to have $300 of their own money, supposedly beyond the nursing home operator's reach. (The amount varies according to state. In Massachusetts, a welfare recipient may have $2,000 of his own. As far as I have been able to discover, few questions have been raised in any state as to who ultimately gets patients' savings if the patient dies at the home, particularly those sums belonging to patients without families and those with savings accounts whose passbooks are held by the nursing home operator.)

bank accounts of Riverside patients, and review three in depth before our research was called off. How many such accounts actually existed we were never to know. After our third visit, Strauss prevented Paul Lilley and me from returning to Riverside. And I received a call from a worker in the county welfare department, telling me she had informed her department that Max Strauss had a clean record.

Before our research was so abruptly terminated, we had discerned a pattern of operations in the three bank accounts we had been able to study. All three showed one substantial deposit—a lump-sum, retroactive Social Security payment to the patient. We saw that when patients received such retroactive benefits, Max Strauss would open bank accounts for them, becoming the self-appointed protector of their funds. He had not legally sought or secured a power of attorney or rights of guardianship to legitimize his name on those books; he had made no legal appeal for the use of his patients' funds. The patients themselves did not make withdrawals from their accounts; at least one patient did not even realize he had such an account.

As recipients of the lump-sum, retroactive payments, the patients (wittingly or not) enjoyed a change of status at Riverside. They were reclassified from welfare recipients to the more costly role of private patients, and the charges for their care rose considerably. Strauss would reimburse himself from their bank accounts until the accounts were depleted. The scraps of paper in their folders showed how these "private" patients were charged for goods and services that in some instances they did not receive. For example, regular withdrawals of $10 were made from one patient's account, supposedly to pay for a physician's visits, but the physician's office had no record of some of those visits.

One case history, illustrating all these activities, was that of Harry Marshall, a veteran dispatched to Riverside Nursing Home from a mental hospital. He arrived with approximately $300, which formed the nucleus for a bank account. The account read, "Max and Lillian Strauss, custodians for Harry Marshall." Neither Marshall, the county welfare department, nor the probate court were consulted on Marshall's need for, and choice of, a custodian. Welfare money would make up the difference between Marshall's Social Security pension and the cost of the nursing home care. At the time he entered the home, his Social Security benefits had not been processed. At some time, therefore, Social Security would send a retroactive lump-sum benefit accompanying the first monthly check. Strauss discovered that Marshall was a veteran entitled to a veteran's pension, for which he then applied. As with the Social Security benefit, the first veteran's check would be accompanied by a retroactive payment. Within a few months of his placement at Riverside, Marshall received approximately $3,000 in retroactive payments and monthly pension checks totaling over $200. Marshall was no longer entitled to public assistance; as a private patient, he had now to use his savings for nursing home care until he had only $300 left, and again became eligible for Medicaid.

That was Strauss's story; the bankbook told another. With the passbook in hand, Lilley went down each withdrawal, asking the reason. Strauss, fumbling through the folder, would find the scrap of paper on which were written figures not always corresponding to the total withdrawn. From the first withdrawal on December 22, 1966, through to June 21, 1968, the entries were questioned. "Max, on July 3, 1967, you drew out $143.32. Why?" The slip of paper found, Strauss replied, "$121.05 was for nursing care, $10.00 for the physician, Dr. Schlitt, $12.27 for medications."

"July 17, Max, you drew out $1,500. Why?"

"Well, I put it back on the nineteenth."

No scrap of paper could be found for this withdrawal— Strauss had borrowed it for his own use. He calmly explained it away as money needed for the payroll. On August 11 he withdrew another $1,100, repaid on the twenty-first.

He again said he had only "borrowed" the money. In spite of Strauss's glib answers, Marshall's bank balance had been reduced to less than $300.

When the first retroactive payment came, Marshall became a private patient. The same room that he had occupied the day before for the $200 welfare rate now cost $125 per month more. Twice after the first increase, Strauss raised the charges. Having set the rate himself, he then paid himself by drawing money, as Marshall's custodian, from the patient's account.

Marshall's account was drained each month for services such as haircuts given by Strauss and taxicab rides to hospitals that were actually rides in Strauss's own car, billed at cab rates with added hourly charges for Strauss's time. The slips of paper showed money withdrawn to pay the physician, although the physician's records deny his receiving that amount. The amount of $84.56 was withdrawn for a hospital treatment for which care the hospital had no record. And while Strauss drew from Marshall's account amounts ranging from $3.75 to $51.00 a month to cover medications as a private patient, Marshall was receiving medications under two publicly supported programs: Medicaid and the Veterans drug program. There were never any official receipts for the drugs charged against Marshall.

Marshall's account was tapped not only for room and board and nursing care at rates ranging up to $125 a month above the amount being paid by most patients, but it also paid around $800 for sundries for which there were no receipts. All decisions to pay and buy were made by Strauss; Marshall was labeled by Strauss an incompetent.

Harry Marshall's health seemed to flourish in inverse ratio to his bank balance: as the balance skidded (making him eligible again for welfare), he suddenly needed no more expensive "cab" rides for care—or, indeed, little else at all from Max Strauss. He was again charged the lower welfare rate for his unchanged accommodations until, when I reported to the Veterans Administration on his rifled bank account, a guardian was appointed for him, and he was moved out of Riverside Nursing Home to the veterans hospital.

How many other bank accounts were raided by Max Strauss? As I have noted, we were cut off from a full answer to that question.

We did, however, learn of Mary Pownall, who arrived at Riverside in January 1968. By the end of the month she was asking to be sent home, believing herself well enough to manage without the "skilled nursing care" of Riverside. But two formidable obstacles stayed her departure. Because of a total and permanent disability she received a lump-sum Social Security check amounting to $572, and thereafter received two monthly pension checks. With these, the die was cast for Mary Pownall. Max Strauss opened a bank account for her, classified her as a private patient at the $12 daily rate, and when she persistently asked to be released, told her she would have to wait for a doctor to sign her out. She waited for a doctor who never did arrive. Meanwhile, the Riverside operator continued to accept Medicaid checks for her care, and by adding these to her bank balance, prolonged her time as a "private" patient. (Subsequently, Max Strauss refunded these Medicaid payments to the state, but not until after Mrs. Pownall had left his nursing home.) At the end of three months her bank balance, although augmented by the Medicaid checks, had shriveled to $84.43, and, still without having been visited by a physician, Mary Pownall was permitted to go home.

Miss Vanderpool was one who beat the system. When, as aides recounted, she received a lump-sum retroactive Social Security payment of $1,700, Max Strauss proposed to her that she open a bank account with himself as custodian. Her powers of judgment unimpaired, Miss Vanderpool rejected the operator's proposal and opened an account under her own control. Forthwith, she was ejected from Riverside

Nursing Home, whose professional care she had officially been classified as needing. Strauss simply called a taxi and summarily moved her to an apartment. He did not choose, however, to forward her mail, and confessed that he opened two bank statements addressed to her that arrived after she left. His explanation was simple: he was curious. (He also picked up $552 from the state for her care after her departure.)

Residents at the Riverside Nursing Home served as unknowing vehicles for cheating of other kinds made feasible for the operator because of the complexity of the administration and the monitoring of Medicare and Medicaid. The case of one patient, Miss Anna George, some of whose story I presented to the federal grand jury considering the record of Max Strauss, exemplifies these potentials.

Miss George was not a senile elderly person but suffered a chronic illness. She was ambulatory, capable of taking care of herself and of handling her own money. Her sister, who visited her weekly, followed Miss George's illness, aware that she was paying for services often not needed. Many of these extra services were rendered only after Medicare became law, opening up a new source of money for vendors of services.

In many states, including Ohio, Medicaid reimbursements to a nursing home patient are suspended while that patient is hospitalized, because his hospital expenses are covered by Medicare. Because two different organizations are involved—Medicare and Medicaid—duplicate payments are exceedingly difficult to trace and police.

The listing of Medicaid reimbursements for individual patients appears on computer printouts, large sheets listing all health-care payments to nursing homes, doctors, pharmacists, ambulance companies, and the like. The printout on Miss George reveals these details of her story for one year:

1. Medicare paid for her hospital care for the same nineteen days Medicaid paid for her care as a patient at

Riverside Nursing Home, despite her absence from the nursing home.

2. When, later, she was discharged from Riverside Max Strauss picked up another six days' coverage for her as one of his patients. This time he misstated the date of her discharge.

3. The government paid for 93 days' care for her in an extended-care facility at a higher rate than at Riverside. Miss George claimed she received no additional attention there— nor did she need it.

4. A physician charged $300 for her care in the extended-care facility, although she claims she was not even examined—that he merely stopped at her door three times.

5. During one six-month period, the records show her receiving twenty-one different drugs, five of them ordered only once—although Medicaid records show she had no physician's care during that period. During approximately a 95 days at Riverside, Medicaid paid for 3,061 pills for her.

Eight other cases uncovered in the Riverside investigation gave evidence of the kind of double payment made for Miss George by Medicaid and Medicare. In most of these cases, the hospital where Medicare paid for a patient who was also being paid for at Riverside by Medicaid did not even have a record of the patient's case, compounding the confusion. Time after time, records of Medicare, hospitals, and nursing homes fail to harmonize, nor does anyone try to reconcile them.

In all these ways, Anna George became the means whereby a nursing home owner and various purveyors of services were enabled to extract unjustified payments from the state and federal governments. Taxpayers paid twice, or paid for services of dubious need, but not even the state auditor could easily have detected that fact. No proof was required that the services were needed, much less proof that such services had in fact been provided.

The bills submitted to the state frequently do not list

information such as dates of service, name of physician requesting the service, destinations of ambulance trips. Under such a vague system of reporting, it is almost impossible to check specific bills. Charges by vendors arc not required to be sent to the paying agency by any reasonable deadline, and frequently these bills arrive long after the service has supposedly been rendered. Thus, a doctor may submit his bill any time within a year; meanwhile, charges for drugs for that same patient may be submitted, and the records as presently constituted cannot show if the drugs were ordered before or after the patient was seen by the physician.

Overlapping of Medicare and Medicaid coverage and resultant abuses have been attested to in other states. For example, the California Department of Justice reviewed Medicare and Medi-Cal (that state's Medicaid program) and affirmed that duplicate payments frequently occur. The report charged that some homes had arrangements with hospitals to transfer patients from nursing homes to hospitals for three days so the homes might qualify anew for a period of Medicare coverage at higher rates for the patients, Hospitals were paid for unnecessary X rays, laboratory tests, and so on ordered by cooperative physicians serving nursing home patients; their cooperation sometimes extended to ordering unnecessary hospitalization. The report stated that some nursing homes charged for patients who had died or been discharged from the home prior to the period charged for, and it referred to kickbacks paid to nursing homes by purveyors of other services that often were not needed, Gradually, investigations in state upon state are bringing forth evidence that Max Strauss's methods are widespread in the nursing home industry.

Payment for services never performed requires arrangements between the nursing home and its suppliers, especially the physicians. (This topic is taken up in detail in Chapter 8.) Strauss took over Riverside in the fall of 1966.

Until June of 1968 he used one physician exclusively. (He also had his favorite pharmacy, ambulance company, funeral home, laboratory, and podiatrist.) Of all the Medicaid-supported patients in the home during that time, the printout shows that the physician saw only five, and those five only once. Nevertheless, he willingly signed the death certificates of patients he apparently had not seen, stating causes of their deaths, the period of time during which he had seen them, and the date of his last visits to them. And he prescribed drugs for patients without, according to the Medicaid records, ever seeing them.

The favorite pharmacy regularly billed the state for medication. The records reveal a haphazard history of new prescriptions added, old prescriptions dropped, one drug ordered twice in a month, then skipped for several months, then reordered without any pattern of reasonable use. The records show that the state is purchasing too many drugs, too wide a variety for each patient, and prescription drugs without evidence of a physician's examination. Perhaps the drugs are never sent, or are diverted to other outlets, or perhaps patients are callously drugged with any medications the nurses choose.

Laboratory work charged to the government for Riverside patients cost many hundreds of dollars. Laboratory work must by law be ordered by a physician, and the findings must be interpreted by a physician. During the period I checked, no patient, with two exceptions, saw a physician before or after the laboratory work had been done. The laboratory may never have done the work; the work may never have been needed, and if performed, never used.

Medicaid cheerfully paid the ambulance company for transporting patients without any record of where the patient was delivered. The suspicion arises that the trip was never taken. Furthermore, the amount charged by the same ambulance company varies for the same trip, suggesting that the charge bears little connection to the reasonable cost.

The podiatrist came with a monotonous regularity until the Medicaid program refused to cover podiatrist services unless ordered by a physician. Whereupon the podiatrist ceased going to Riverside, immediately.

While he was pursuing his various hustles, Max Strauss was, like so many other operators, complaining that government payments were so low that he had to cut corners in order to make ends meet. He admitted that one way of trimming costs at Riverside was to limit expenditures for food to sixty-nine cents per patient daily. Strauss acknowledged that he sought bargains in food purchases: "Sure, I buy day-old bread, cheaper cuts of meat, dented and damaged canned goods, spotted and soft peaches for 50 cents a basket, and tomatoes that may be bruised. How else can you keep food costs down?" An aide at Riverside gave a more colorful account:

> The cook has taken hams, bacon, and wieners and thrown them on Strauss's desk because of their smell, and refused to prepare them. . . .
>
> Often the cook has thrown away whole baskets of tomatoes Strauss purchased at the market for stewing because they were unfit to eat.
>
> And sometimes the cook almost flips a coin to decide whether she should use the contents of a damaged, rusted, and bulging can.

On the West Coast, last summer, I learned about another nursing home operator who was, if anything, even more ingenious than Max Strauss in procuring food "bargains" for the helpless ones under his wing.

He was Herbert Cook, family man, involved citizen, a former retailer with a master's degree (though not in the health field), whose future seemed most promising. From his modest entry into the nursing home business in 1959, he had risen to become the owner of four homes large enough to accommodate a total of approximately one thousand patients. His total assets are reportedly in excess of $2 million; his net worth is estimated in the court record as in the range of $750,000, and his monthly income is $10,000.

But Cook slipped on the ladder to success. It had been his habit to purchase groceries at a place called McCoy's Market; but a state's witness in a case against Cook testified that, because Cook was delinquent in paying his bills at McCoy's, the market had refused further business with him. Thereupon, Cook allegedly approached an employee at the market with the proposition that he, on his own, sell the nursing home owner eggs and coffee at "reasonable prices." The employee reportedly agreed, and according to his own testimony, delivered twenty-one cases of eggs and eight cases of coffee to two of the four homes each week, for which he was paid by cash and by check, with an entry for a nonexistent company accounting for the transaction.

Most of those eggs were what are called "checks and dirties," which, by California law, may not be served in nursing homes because of their substandard quality. Some of Cook's fortune was thus amassed by buying inferior food and serving it to patients, aware that what was served was substandard—so aware, in fact, that he ordered these items not to be delivered around the time the inspectors were to visit his homes.

It was not, however, feeding rejected food to his patients that got Cook in trouble with the law. What did was the fact that the food was stolen. Charged with accepting stolen goods, he was fined $1,500 and sentenced to a term of six months in the county jail—subsequently commuted to a work furlough—and placed on probation for an additional eighteen months. Cook appealed for a revocation or at least reduction of this probation period; his lawyer was Murray Chotiner, a long-time adviser and associate of Richard Nixon, and a special counsel to the President during Mr.

Nixon's first term in office. The court, however, declared that it had already made concessions "all along this line," and turned the appeal down.

Max Strauss had other ways of augmenting his income. Like Eugene Woods before him, Strauss intercepted and cashed Social Security checks addressed to his patients. This was inevitable, for the Social Security check is such an easy target that no hustler in the nursing home business could be expected to pass it up. It provides a steady source of extra income with virtually no risk of being caught. To flush out evidence of fraud in the handling of Social Security checks is made all but impossible by the rule of confidentiality protecting such payments. The Social Security Administration maintains that its recipients have a right to privacy. Ironically, this position prevents exposure of abuses of the system, and gives nursing home operators the dangerous right to decide, on their own, which patients can or cannot handle their own affairs.

This freedom to appraise the patients' mental and physical powers had permitted the operator of Riverside Nursing Home to decide that all but five of his patients were unable to endorse their own Social Security checks. Some former employees described the endorsing procedure followed by Max Strauss. Their description is similar to that of Mary Burrows, the employee who got into trouble by complaining about Eugene Woods.

Usually, a number of checks for patients would arrive in the same mail. The operator would open the envelopes, place all checks face down on a clipboard, and have an employee sign them as a witness, although there was no signature to be witnessed. Later, Max Strauss would endorse each check with the name of the home and an X, presumably made by the patient. The employees could not know to whom the checks had been paid, nor in what amounts—a circumstance that fed their suspicions that they were signing as witnesses checks not only for patients who could, themselves, sign, but also for individuals who were not even patients at Riverside. To those few patients adjudged able to sign for themselves, the checks were presented as they were to the employees—face down on a clipboard, with the patients required to sign without being able to see the amount for which the checks were written.

That this method of blind endorsement is accepted by the Social Security Administration opens several advantages to dishonest operators: patients' resources may be understated so that the operator can collect more from Medicaid, with no witness to the understatement; retroactive payments may be concealed from patients; checks received at homes for patients temporarily absent—those hospitalized, for example—may be cashed; checks for patients who have died, and checks for patients housed elsewhere, may be cashed. No government agency has demanded a rigorous accounting of the disposition of Social Security checks, though they go out to every nursing home in the country for virtually every patient.

To understate a patient's resources—income from Social Security, private pensions, investments, or contributions from families—is against the law. The operator has the responsibility to report the correct amount of the patient's income to the state. Max Strauss was found to understate patients' income, to his own benefit, both before and after he became the subject of widespread publicity. Because of his repeated understatement of patients' income, Strauss was forced to make refunds in 1969 of various petty sums, though the refunds did not cover the entire periods during which patients' resources were understated. The fact that these refunds were made at all indicate that, at least for a time, Max Strauss was subjected to close scrutiny by the county caseworker—but he was never penalized.

Ohio nursing homes are not alone in their practice of understating patients' resources. The state of California recovered $21,664 from one home alone in 1971 for misstatements, $6,000 of which was of patients' income. The state could not classify the action as fraudulent, since so many people are involved in the process of determining a patient's income that it is nearly impossible to prove that such miscalculations result from intent rather than from clerical errors.

Checks for retroactive payments are a particular temptation to acquisitive operators. One is the lump sum sent to a person newly eligible for Social Security; the amount may be substantial if, as often happens, the person did not apply when he first became eligible. Increased benefits are allotted—often beginning with a check for a retroactive sum-to women who as wives have received Social Security through their husbands and as widows become entitled to larger benefits. In his reporting to the state, Max Strauss understated the amounts of some widows' increased Social Security benefits. When one of his blind patients was widowed, Strauss claimed that the amount of her retroactive check was $106 less than it actually was.

Another source of retroactive payments is an increase in Social Security benefits voted by Congress for all recipients. Who polices the disposition of retroactive raises to patients? The nursing home operators. The Social Security agency depends solely upon them for the honest disposition of these sometimes considerable sums.

A Social Security increase should be reflected in lower bills to Medicaid, since it is Medicaid that makes up the difference between the patient's Social Security check and the nursing home charges. The operators typically take their time in reporting the change. Three months after the first checks went out under the 1972 increase, many Ohio nursing homes had yet to report any change in their patients' income.

Official interest in what happens to the retroactive checks appears to be slight. In 1971, for example, all homes in Ohio received a letter from the state director of welfare advising them that forthcoming retroactive checks should be added to the patients' personal expense funds—those funds which are everywhere most vulnerable to theft, protected by almost no official monitoring. A cynic would have viewed that letter as an invitation to steal.

Even death does not end the hustles in the nursing home business. Social Security claims to have effective safeguards against the cashing of checks received after the beneficiary has died. Funeral homes, for instance, have agreed to notify the agency of the deaths of those having Social Security numbers. Death benefits will not be paid until that last check has been returned to Social Security, supposedly giving the funeral homes an incentive to report accurately and promptly. However, an undertaker, in collusion with a nursing home operator, can misstate the dates of deaths, thereby earning an illicit bonus for the operator. In return, the operator might favor the establishment with as much business as he can send him.

Such an alliance was said to have existed between Max Strauss and one funeral home. This suspicion was voiced by Riverside employees who, upon the deaths of some patients, were instructed to send the bodies to that specific undertaker before notifying the family (if any) of the death. The advantage to a funeral home of being so chosen can be seen in the fact that if the family of a deceased person has not claimed his death benefits within ninety days, the funeral home can file for the benefits, supposedly to cover funeral expenses. Since approximately half of all nursing home patients have no immediate families, funeral homes can, through being favored by nursing homes, become regular claimants for death benefits that can total as much as $255. (By contrast, Cuyahoga County only pays $75 for the burial expenses of a general relief recipient.)

The responses to the newspaper revelations of the Riverside scandal took several forms. Former employees came forth to voice their stored-up complaints; families emerged briefly to recount their own stories of theft and abuse; welfare officials were agitated. And the United States government, through the Department of Health, Education, and Welfare and the Veterans Administration, called for an investigation. The director of Cuyahoga County welfare recommended, at the height of the storm, the revocation of Max Strauss's nursing home license. That license was never revoked. Riverside Nursing Home, operated by Max Strauss, is in business today, and the county welfare department continues to place patients there.

According to protocol, that county department was to conduct the investigation for HEW. The department found that "a few overpayments" had been made to Strauss, but assured the regional office of HEW that all refunds had been made. Because Max Strauss paid back some of the amounts he had taken, he enjoyed total forgiveness.

But HEW, in an unusual show of interest, believed it should know the number of refunds and the reason each was made. It called upon the state of Ohio to check these out, and the state welfare department, in response, sent a medical consultant, who had lately submitted a favorable report on Riverside, to return to the home and check her own findings. She found herself to have been correct in the first place. The state health department, which had approved Riverside as a skilled nursing home, sent an inspector to check on the newspaper's reports concerning inedible food served there. The person chosen by the department for this task had reported a few months previously that Riverside was not in complete compliance with regulations. Dispatched on this repeat investigation, she found that the home was now in compliance. Strauss was in the clear.

Prodded by agitated Ohio congressmen, Social Security then sent in to Cleveland one of the ten investigators who then policed the entire Social Security program throughout the country. His investigative methods consisted of these steps: (1) he talked to some patients at Riverside to get what he dubbed a "layman's view" of their actual ability to endorse their own checks; (2) he talked to Max Strauss, assuring him of his constitutional rights; (3) he reported that he felt Strauss was "shopping around for an explanation on the Social Security checks."

Nothing having come of that "investigation," the agency took one step beyond sending its man to Riverside. It examined a sample of nursing homes around the country to determine how its checks were being endorsed. The study revealed that in each of the homes examined some 85 percent of the patients' checks were endorsed with an X—convincing evidence to me that the Woods-Strauss methods are generally practiced in U.S. nursing homes.

This alarming finding led to some soul-searching by Social Security officials. Commissioner Robert M. Ball explained the agency's reaction to Ohio Congressman Charles Vanik, who had taken an interest in the Riverside exposé, by saying: "We are reviewing our internal processes to see what changes can be made which will build into our processes the greatest protection for Social Security beneficiaries." But nothing further occurred. Evidently the effort of change was adjudged greater than the benefit such change might bring.

In the course of all this, I was told by a Secret Service agent that the United States Attorney views fraudulent cashing of Social Security checks by nursing homes as "nuisance cases" and does not prosecute. Even when evidence is found of wrongful cashing of checks over a considerable period, I was informed, the government will settle the case on a return of only part of the amount wrongfully taken.

Thereafter, the Department of Health, Education, and Welfare abandoned its investigation of Max Strauss's nursing home. The whole futile grinding of gears had taken six months.

But all was not yet lost. The Veterans Administration, having discovered the misuse of their payments to Harry Marshall, had asked for an investigation of fraud on the part of Max Strauss. Under this pressure from the VA, the United States district attorney in Cleveland, Benjamin Stuplinsky, brought the case to the federal grand jury for a hearing.

I appeared before that jury, testifying for four hours. The federal prosecutor seemed to be driven by one overwhelming concern: to remind the jury that the county prosecutor was the one who rightfully should be involved in the case. Between sessions and after the hearings, he professed sympathy with me. However, he failed to use his powers of subpoena to obtain the data necessary to establish a true case—the checks admittedly signed by Max Strauss without the patients' knowledge. During the investigation, the regional branch of the Ohio Nursing Home Association expressed its support of Max Strauss. By going to the defense of one of its members, without looking into the documentation underlying the news articles, the association showed the uncritical cooperation binding nursing homes into a group for mutual defense.

Max Strauss was not indicted. That was 1968. In 1970 I received an unexpected call from a person in the Justice Department's Fraud Division in Washington who said he wished to reassure me that the case against Max Strauss was "still open." One year later, in 1971, I called the office of the new district attorney for Cuyahoga County to learn what, if anything, had happened. An assistant attorney explained that the office had concluded it did not have a case. Of the interest-free loans made by Max Strauss to himself from patients' accounts, he declared that since the money had been returned there was "no problem ... no case." The attorney saw a silver lining in the whole situation: the investigation, he was convinced, had reformed Max Strauss.

Perhaps so—anything can happen.* But if a swindling

* And then again, perhaps not. On August 31, 1973, Congressman James V. Stanton of Ohio wrote the .state nursing home division requesting an investigation of Max Strauss's Riverside Nursing Home. "From what has been reported by my constituents and other sources, there appears to be good

nursing home operator decides to go straight, it is not because of anything our governments do. Nothing in the actions taken by the agencies to whom we entrust our old people and our tax dollars has succeeded in preventing their exploitation by unscrupulous operators. In these circumstances, it is no surprise that so many operators practice the swindles we have been describing. What is perhaps surprising is that there are some honest people in a business that virtually offers a license to steal.

Max Strauss and Eugene Woods are representative of one kind of nursing home hustler. I have chosen these two because I was intimately familiar with their cases, but each time anyone bothers to investigate the industry, their counterparts are found all over the nation. Their methods of hustling, the means they use to maximize government revenue and minimize service, are fairly easy to understand: this kind of swindling has been around a long time. More recently, however, the industry has been invaded by a different breed of swindler—the financial manipulators—and compared to them, nickel-and-dimers like Woods and Strauss are small fry. The newcomers are big operators. Their methods of taking our money are exceedingly complex, difficult to detect, and in many cases legal: the threat of jail is even more remote for these operators than it is for the old-timers. In the following chapters we will meet some of these newcomers to the nursing home game.

---

reason to have this nursing home checked out," Stanton wrote. According to the Cleveland Department of Public Health, the complaints "concerned odors, dirty premises, flies and patients fearing the nursing staff."

5

Owners:
The Secret Sharers

WHO OWNS AMERICAN NURSING HOMES? This is a surprisingly difficult question to answer, and many of the most sophisticated swindles in the business arc hidden from public view by the secrecy that protects nursing home ownership.

Government agencies that regulate nursing homes do not know who owns the homes they regulate, for the good reason that they have never tried to find out this most basic information. When I set out to uncover for myself the information my government was unwilling to gather, I found, by piecing together bits of evidence from various records, enough to become convinced that many nursing home owners have excellent reasons for seeing to it that their ownership remains secret.

Nursing home administrators must be licensed, and their identity is therefore no secret. Operators must also be identified, but the operator is just the person or company that runs the business, not the owner of the physical plant, the land and buildings and equipment. The owner is the one who makes most of the decisions and collects most of the profits. In the old clays, before the Hood of government money, most operators also owned the property. But the trend now is for the operator and owner to be different—at least on paper. This is especially true of the smart financial hustlers who have invaded the industry in recent years. Typically, my investigation of ownership turned up this situation: the operator was identified, while the owner was a deliberately vague entity who, when closer examination was possible, turned out to be the operator himself, or someone close to him, wearing a different set of hats. In other cases the owner is someone who will never appear on any record as connected with the nursing home business.

Why these subterfuges?

Profit is the main, though by no means the only, reason for concealed ownership. There are a couple of basic patterns in this part of the game. In some cases the goal is to get a higher reimbursement rate from Medicaid or Medicare, while in others the object is to avoid paying income taxes; but in all cases the ultimate victim of the con is the taxpayer.

Here is one way it's done. If you own and operate a nursing home, you set up another corporation with other names as officers, ostensibly unrelated to you, and sell the home to that corporation. You may sell it at an inflated price, which has the effect of transforming profits into capital gains, taxed at a lower rate. Then you rent it back at an inflated rent. You may also buy goods and services from that corporation, or others you set up, all on the surface unrelated to you, and you pay more than fair value for what you buy from those corporations. The purpose of all those maneuvers is to shift profits out of the nursing home to some other place you also control. One reason for that shift is to help sustain the case that nursing homes arc underpaid by government—excess profits might undercut that argument. Another is that nursing homes, being mainly supported by government, have to reveal more information than the related corporations. If you are going to put yourself on the payroll as a "consultant" and your family on as "officers," and charge those trips to Florida as business expenses, it is better not to have all that gravy appearing on the books of the nursing home. (As always, the patient is victimized. Purchasing at excessive prices inevitably puts a squeeze on the nursing home budget, at the expense of patient care. In fact, patients appear to be just as neglected in the homes run by the financial manipulators as they are in the homes of the more old-fashioned operators like Eugene Woods. The explanation in both cases is the same: profit.)

In theory, that kind of maneuvering is banned by the principle of arm's-length negotiation. Costs like rentals are acceptable at face value (by tax and regulatory agencies) only if they were negotiated at arm's length—that is, between two unrelated parties that are not in collusion. In practice, however, nursing home hustlers are .smarter and more motivated than government investigators, and it is pretty easy, by rapid shuffling of properties, to conceal the trail from both the regulators and the Internal Revenue. So I have found that nursing homes are forever changing "ownership" on paper while remaining in the control of the same people.

Another reason for this fast shuffle is to avoid repaying money illegitimately collected. As noted in the last chapter, nursing home operators are sometimes called upon to return government money they have taken for patients who were dead or not in the home. If the home changes ownership, the government will not pursue the new owners for the refund, so if the owner has been caught in a substantial overcharge, it may be worth switching owners for that reason alone. Besides avoiding repayment, a concealed owner can also avoid being cited for violations in his home. When the government inspector comes around with a demand that this or that violation be corrected, there is no one on the scene except the administrator. He can be told what has to be done, but it is the owner alone who can pay for the necessary improvements, and if the inspector does not know who the owner is, he is hardly likely to find him and make him comply. Honest inspectors have often told me that concealed ownership multiplies the problems of enforcement.

Concealed ownership has still another set of advantages. Some people have good reason to keep their status as owners out of the public eye. If, for example, they are putting heavy mortgages on their nursing homes to finance other enterprises—what is commonly known as "pyramiding"—they may not want government to know what they are doing with its money. Sometimes a conflict of interest is being concealed, a conflict that may involve a political figure eager to get in on nursing home profits but not wanting it known that he is in a position to influence the regulation of the home. Or it may be a doctor who steers patients to what is his own business. Some owners may not want the public to know how many homes they control. Finally, there is the persistent rumor that the Mafia has gotten into nursing homes. I have heard this suspicion stated by officials in several states (Michigan, Massachusetts, New Jersey, Connecticut, Louisiana, and Ohio), but as yet I have seen no hard evidence. In New Jersey, a noted Mafioso, Simone Rizzo de Cavalcante ("Sam the Plumber"), said of a Plain-field nursing home, "I got money in there," while explaining that he did not want a labor union organizing that home (according to an FBI phone tap quoted in the *New York Times*). I checked the records, but of course his name does not appear.

Not only the name of Sam the Plumber, but many far more important ones are missing from the records. Indeed, I am convinced that if we had a list of the dozen most powerful people in the nursing home industry, most of them would not be found in the records as they are now kept, or they would appear in a way that did not reflect their true importance. Finding out who owns nursing homes—who makes the decisions and who rakes in the profits—is an extremely difficult undertaking. I have spent many months poring over records of various kinds in an effort to track down the owners of certain homes. Sometimes I have failed, and when I have succeeded, it was because I was more persistent in following the owner's tracks than he was in covering them.

The case of Bernard Bergman and the Towers Nursing Home in New York City is a good example of such an investigation. Dr. Bergman's story illustrates many of the effects of concealed ownership. Although he admitted to me that he owns nursing homes in five states and is a major stockholder in a large, "publicly owned" chain, Medic-Home Enterprises, the true extent of his holdings does not appear on the public record.

Much of what I learned about Bergman's enterprises came from information the company was required to submit to the Securities and Exchange Commission in order to get permission to sell its stock to the public. I also interviewed Dr. Bergman and a financial officer of his corporation in the offices of Medic-Home Enterprises, Inc., on the forty-second floor of a building on Broadway in Manhattan.

By the time we met, I had been following the growth of his Medic-Home Enterprises for some time (in the SEC files and through interviews with government personnel), and I knew it to be an expanding business. Dr. Bergman told me he owns a number of homes in his own right beyond those included in the Medic-Home chain, of which he is chairman of the board. He did not name the homes nor tell me where they were located. He did, however, say—an ironic statement, in view of what I later learned—that he ran his own nursing homes separately from Medic-Home because he would never allow himself to be involved in any agreement that was not the result of arm's-length negotiation.

Later in the interview, when Dr. Bergman had to leave, his financial vice-president, Mr. Marvin Wolfe, continued. He expressed his hope that he would not "live to see the day when nursing homes cannot operate under high standards and still make money." Dr. Bergman, he said, has made a lot of money and is a very wealthy man. Besides Medic-Home Enterprises, he runs nursing homes under the name of National Hospitals and Institutional Builders. Medic-Home leases equipment from National Hospitals—a fact that is publicly known only because Medic-Home, as a public corporation, was required to submit copies of the leases to the SEC. Dr. Bergman had not mentioned this leasing activity to me— nor another lease involving the Towers Nursing Home in Manhattan, which had originally aroused my interest in him. And Dr. Bergman's activities in the field are not limited to ownership and leasing: he also has a construction company that builds nursing homes to meet his personal specifications.

By the time I left the Medic-Home office, my questions had been answered with apparent candor. But baffling facts remained in the Medic-Home story. One was the curious leasing arrangements on the Towers Nursing Home. The events occurred in the following sequence and are doubtless no more confusing to the reader than to a regulatory agency trying to figure out what was going on:

1. In 1958 the Bogardus Realty Corporation signed a thirty-eight-page lease, renting the Towers to one Anne Weiss. Buried on page 36 of the lease was the information that the Towers had been deeded to Bogardus Realty by Anne Weiss on the same day she signed the lease. (In later years the name of Bogardus Realty disappears from the record, and the owner of the property is listed as Towers Associates, a firm in which Anne Weiss is a partner.)

2. In 1965 the lease on the Towers was purchased from Anne Weiss for $1,026,000 by Liberty House of New York, Inc. Liberty House is a wholly owned subsidiary of Dr. Bergman's Medic-Home Enterprises. The rental payable under the lease was $10,833 per month, plus real estate and water taxes. Subsequently (on an unspecified later date), Liberty subleased the property back to Anne Weiss, who agreed to pay a rental of $25,000 per month (a figure that rose to $30,000 per month in 1967 when fifty beds were

added to the home). By that time, Medic-Home Enterprises had offered its stock to the public; its prospectus said of the Towers: "The lease price" to Liberty (more than $1 million) "and the sublease rental" (an increase from approximately $11,000 per month to $25,000 per month) "were determined by negotiation."

Who owned the Towers? Licensing personnel in New York City were somewhat vague on this point. The lease was held, they said, by one Anne Weiss, who operated the home with a partner. Since she was merely the lessee, her responsibility was not well defined, and the owner—whoever he was—could not be coerced into action when violations occurred. Dr. Ray Trussell, then commissioner of the New York City hospitals, and who had jurisdiction over nursing homes, declared he could find no proven ownership interest in the Towers on the part of Dr. Bergman.

The fact was that Anne Weiss, the lessee, was Mrs. Bernard Bergman.

I discovered this information in the 1968 prospectus and exhibits of Medic-Home Enterprises, filed with the Securities and Exchange Commission when Medic-Home offered its stock to the public. Dr. Bergman, as an officer of the company, was required to state his interest in corporate transactions. Since Anne Weiss was known to be a participant in the intricate lease arrangements for the Towers, her relationship to Dr. Bergman had to be admitted. That relationship, which was ostensibly unknown to local authorities, was to be found in public files at the SEC.

What was reality in this tangle? On paper, the Towers was controlled by Anne Weiss (the operator), Liberty House (owner of the lease), and Towers Associates (owner of the property). No Bergman there. But Anne Weiss is Bergman's wife, Liberty House is owned by a company in which Bergman is the major stockholder, and Anne Weiss is a partner in Towers Associates. Another way of stating the facts is that the Towers is owned and operated by Dr. and Mrs. Bergman.

Why, then, does Dr. Bergman go to such lengths to avoid being identified? Only he knows the full answer, but the record suggests several possibilities. During one of the changes of name, the rent was more than doubled, from $10,833 a month to $25,000, although the value of the property remained the same. If this could be accepted as an "arm's-length" deal between unrelated persons, the basis would be laid for income tax savings and for raising the rates to patients. Certainly the rates did go up, from $350 a month in 1965 to $704 in 1972. Potential investors who read the Medic-Home prospectus, reading the rental figure and the statement that most patients were on Medicaid, would get the impression that the government was guaranteeing the company $25,000 a month for the Towers, increasing the company's income and the value of its stock. (In reality, state officials never allowed the Towers full credit for the rental of $25,000 in setting the home's reimbursement rate.)

Another motive, suggested earlier, has to do with responsibility for the property. In one of her leases, Anne Weiss agreed to make improvements valued at $100,000 within three years. Six years later I visited the Towers, a gloomy old fort of a building on Central Park West, to see if those improvements had been made. One promise was the installation of "automatic window screens." I saw screens that did not fit and others that were patched, and windows with no screens at all; it was summer, and flies were buzzing around the patients. Another promise was a physical therapy room. I did find a room with a makeshift sign—Physical Therapy Room—but inside I saw only one piece of equipment: steps leading up to a platform and down on the other side. That one piece of equipment was pushed against the wall, while most of the room was occupied by two tables obviously used for dining. In short, the promised improvements had been quite blatantly reneged on; yet it was impossible to hold Dr. Bergman himself to account. (It might also be noted in passing, just to show that the Towers is not above the mundane hustles of a Woods or a Strauss, that in 1971 the New York state comptroller cited the home for collecting for 926 days of care for patients who were either dead or discharged.)

From the standpoint simply of concealment, the strategy was also successful, though not permanently. Officials at the New York State Department of Health, which took over regulation of nursing homes from the city in 1967, said it took them "quite a while to figure out" that Anne Weiss was Dr. Bergman's wife. They knew as well, they added, that the Towers was not an isolated case. They are sure that Bergman owns other homes in the New York City area, perhaps a couple of dozen, but his name appears nowhere, though Anne Weiss is listed as operator of several homes besides the Towers in the city, and one in Utica. The same is true of at least two other states where Bergman operates, New Jersey and Florida. When I called the licensing authorities in those states, they said they had no record of his name, though Bergman himself says he owns homes in both states.

Sham arm's-length deals are commonplace in New York, the state officials admit. According to them, the great majority of leases between nursing home operators and owners are in fact deals involving one person masquerading as two in the interests of taking more money away from the taxpayers. New York State's efforts to combat these maneuvers do not seem destined for success. In the case of the Towers, the state in 1972 cut its rental reimbursement from $212,770 to $143,961. (New York reimburses nursing homes for rental under a formula that gives a lower amount if the agreement is held not to have been made at arm's length.) But, as of early 1973, Bergman's lawyer had already written the state claiming that the Towers lease was arm's length and therefore entitled to a higher rate. So had Towers Associates, the owner of the property, in a letter signed by Anne Weiss. The law is so weak that the state officials at that time thought they would probably have to give in to Bergman's claim that the deal between Mrs. Bergman and Dr. Bergman was between two unrelated parties—and give the Towers more tax money.

The loss to the public, in the case of the Towers alone, is small. Multiplied many times, to take into account all the sham deals with concealed owners all over the nation, the loss to us becomes impressive.

The Towers pattern was repeated later on a larger scale by Medic-Home, Dr. Bergman's chain. In 1972, according to the *Wall Street Journal,* Medic-Home leased out all the homes it owned to one Homer Cunningham, who had just resigned as vice-president of Medic-Home, and to William J. Lemon, a former director.

The operations of Medic-Home give further evidence of the way nursing home ownership is maneuvered to achieve maximum cost to the public. In 1969 Medic-Home bought Care Centers, ten money-losing Florida homes, at what appears to have been an irrationally high price. Medic-Home paid about $4¼ million and assumed the mortgages on the homes, for a total price tag of about $9 million. Ernst and Ernst auditors declared that $3,759,810 of that amount was "in excess of the underlying net assets of Care Centers, Inc.," although, in the guarded language of the profession, the auditors also reported that Medic-Home considered this to be a fair value. The president of Care Centers, R. D. Reed, wrote to his stockholders: "Your attention is respectfully directed to the fact that Medic-Home earned $234,544 for its fiscal year ended September 30, 1968 as contrasted with the *loss of* $684,154 *shown by Care Centers* for its fiscal year ended October 31, 1968." [Emphasis mine.]

What had prompted Medic-Home to purchase, at so

inflated a price, a money-losing group of homes described by *Barron's* as having the "poorest operating record" of fifty leading nursing home chains?

No certain explanation was forthcoming, but some advantages were obvious. In absorbing the Care homes, Medic-Home had placed on them a much higher value than they had previously enjoyed. As a result, Medicare's guaranteed percentage return on equity might be calculated on a much higher figure. Secondly, Medic-Home, as the new proprietor, could elect to use accelerated depreciation in its accounting. As compared to the straight-line method (which provides equal, annual amounts of depreciation over the life of an asset), the accelerated method affords the advantage of charging heavy amounts of depreciation to costs in the early years and smaller amounts in the later years. The amount of profit subject to tax in the early years is thus minimized. (Depreciation, for those who do not understand it, provides tax-free income to property-owning businessmen. Before calculating his profits, he is allowed to deduct from his income an amount that the property theoretically declined in value during the year—even if the value of the property in fact increased. That amount is tax-free income and very valuable.) Obviously, substantial gains may be realized if the properties being depreciated by the accelerated method are promptly disposed of after the first few years.

Other explanations for the move suggest themselves. It might well be that the homes bought by Medic-Home at inflated prices might be used as collateral for new loans. The owners of the Care homes, if they had been reimbursed by Medicare for costs that could later be questioned, might have been glad to get out of the picture, since Medicare does not pursue past owners for refunds. The old owners also got handsome capital gains out of the transaction—and that, indeed, is the clearest benefit in the deal.

In order to find out if the inflated sales price had in fact been used to up the reimbursement rate, I went to Washington to examine the cost figures that nursing homes collecting Medicare are required to submit to the Social Security Administration. I wanted to see what effect the inflated purchase price in 1969 had had on the cost reimbursement figure in 1970. To my surprise, out of ten homes in the Care Centers group organized in 1968 and bought in early 1969 by Medic-Home, only two had submitted cost data by June 1970, and the figures for those two homes only covered the years 1967-1968. That was all the cost information available to Social Security. Thus the agency was paying eight homes for costs on the basis of figures never submitted, and was paying two others in 1970 on the basis of figures submitted for 1968—and thus I could learn nothing about the effect of the sales prices. However, I did learn other interesting things from the figures on those two homes.

Each Social Security file is composed of several pages, each of which is referred to as a schedule. These papers include lists of assets, lists of liabilities, and the computation of return on equity capital. No supportive information is required to accompany these schedules. Those filing the papers were permitted to leave blank the schedule on which a certified public accountant is supposed to testify to the accuracy of the figures. Upon receipt of such incomplete and flimsy material, Social Security has paid out more than a billion dollars.

By comparing the registration statement in the SEC files with the cost schedules submitted to Social Security for the same homes, I found discrepancies that work to the benefit of the owners. When the prospectus claims contradicted the Medicare schedules there seemed to be a reason other than simple error. The Care Center prospectus is aimed at enticing the investor by stressing profit potential. The figures for Medicare are prepared for Social Security and thus stress greater costs.

The prospectus announced a larger number of beds for one of the two homes whose files I examined than the licensed capacity listed with Medicare. The prospectus implied that the entire nursing home was certified for Medicare, but the Medicare schedules show that less than half of each of the facilities was so licensed. (There is, for complex reasons, a financial advantage to licensing only part of the home.) In both these illustrations the investor is misled: the larger the number of beds, the larger the income; and the more Medicare patients in the home, the better the image of the home, since Medicare pays the highest reimbursement and requires the highest standards.

For Medicare purposes, the equity figure was improved. Equity most simply explained is the net remaining after debt is subtracted from the worth of the property. Thus a home worth $500,000 and carrying a mortgage of $400,000 has equity of $100,000. Equity increases if either the worth is increased or the mortgage is decreased, other things remaining the same. If, in the above example, the worth of the home rises to $600,000, or if the mortgage is decreased to $300,000, the effect in either case is to double the equity from $100,000 to $200,000. Whichever method is used, the equity figure on which Medicare reimbursement is based goes up. Care Centers did it by submitting wrong figures either to the SEC or to Medicare.

Ocala Care Center, one of the two homes whose files I studied, presents a good illustration. According to the Care Centers prospectus, the home cost $462,000 for land, building, and equipment. It opened on April 1, 1968. In the schedule submitted to Medicare eight months later, the value of the land, building, and equipment had been increased by the company to $520,000—quite a leap in a few months, especially considering that Care Centers was losing money. The depreciation figure was also immediately improved, since there is more to depreciate on $520,000 than on $462,000.

Additional maneuvers with the equity figure resulted in a score against Medicare. The schedule used to compute the return on equity shows that the owners' original investment was $22,000. Each month the schedule that determines equity lists the owners as allegedly loaning the corporation operating the home an additional amount of money. By October 1968, the last month of the fiscal year, the owners had lent it a total of $105,000. The net result at the end of the fiscal year was that the owners had an equity in the business of $45,000, twice the original amount. The higher equity figure would produce a higher Medicare reimbursement rate. But key questions on the forms relating to equity were left blank, and there is, in these uncertified records, no proof of the transactions that produced the higher equity figure.

The mortgage debt on that home also dropped remarkably fast. In the first year of operation the figures submitted by the owners showed the long-term debt dropping by much more than the payments the home was required to make on its mortgage—a neat trick for a home that was losing money at the time. There is no explanation in the record of how that reduction was achieved.

What is most noteworthy in these records is that two federal agencies, the Securities and Exchange Commission and the Social Security Administration (which administers Medicare), allowed nursing home owners to submit documents that are contradictory, incomplete, and uncertified. Yet it is on the basis of these documents that nursing home stock is offered to the public (in the case of the SEC) and that Medicare reimbursement rates are set (in the case of Social Security).

The government-assured revenue of the nursing homes Medic-Home owned provided it with the base for two brief and rather weird flights into other business ventures. The first was the acquisition of a business called Freezie, variously described as a manufacturer of noncarbonated beverages, soft-drink dispensing machines, and ice-making machines. A second subsidiary was formed, Medic-Home

Leasing Corporation, through which Medic-Home Enterprises branched out into the leasing of helicopters. (Originally it was explained they planned the "remanufacturing" of helicopters for commercial use through acquiring, reconditioning, and assembling helicopter parts.) Charles Dunn, an officer of Freezie, became president of Medic-Home Leasing. Dunn previously had leased equipment to nursing homes.

In its annual report to the stockholders, Medic-Home said of the acquisition of Freezie; "This is the initial step in your company's plans to diversify into related fields in order to meet the growing needs of health care services." Since Freezie beverage dispensers were to be installed "at convenience store or news-stand locations," stockholders might have wondered how nursing home patients would have access to these "health care services." But perhaps the implication was, instead, that the buying of Freezie would relieve some of the company's costs of providing care by adding a profit-generating company.

When Freezie was acquired by Medic-Home, the SEC exhibits showed it to be a profitable business. But during the year following its move into Medic-Home, Freezie, continuing under its former management, suffered a catastrophic reversal: that year, its losses exceeded its earnings of the year before. The records contain no explanation for this sudden reversal, nor for the next surprising move. Limping under a loss of more than $1 million, Freezie was sold back to its former owners, including Charles Dunn, who thereby acquired a new building constructed for Freezie while it was owned by Medic-Home.

Nothing in the record shows what Freezie produced or how it went about doing it. One SEC schedule states that principals in Freezie hold interests in nine of the company's client firms. Five clients are listed with the cities in which they supposedly do business, but not one of those firms appears in the telephone book or city directory of the city named in the SEC schedule—and not one figure on the schedule of operating expenses appears to be for manufacturing anything. In order to accomplish the sales of Freezie's mysterious product, it cost the company in one year $24,000 for travel and entertainment, $19,000 for the company plane and $9,000 for the company boat. Freezie did, however, pick up one new customer as a result of its alliance with Medic-Home. Dr. Bernard Bergman and another officer borrowed $88,000 from their own company to buy some of Freezie's mystery machines.

In the summary of earnings in its 1971 annual report, Medic-Home shows these figures for Freezie: in 1968, earnings of $276,386; in 1969, earnings of $452,520; and in 1970, a loss of $1,004,053. That same year the second subsidiary, Medic-Home Leasing Corporation, which in 1969 had earnings of $45,444, turned around and produced a loss of $34,815.

It is peculiar that government-supported nursing homes can be used to finance ventures into the helicopter business and the Freezie business—whatever that business actually was. It is equally peculiar that both those businesses could so quickly be switched from the profit to the loss column.

In addition, examples of the transfers of ownership and changing of costs turned up when I examined figures collected by the Connecticut Hospital Commission in its investigation of nursing home costs. One case involved associates of Joseph Kosow, the Boston-based nursing home financier who is the subject of the next chapter. A sixty-bed home, the Forestville—one of the few in Connecticut operating at a loss—then included among its owners Norman Geller, the CPA in Joseph Kosow's office. The owners' investment was $1,000—little more than i percent of the worth of the asset—indicating the existence of one or more mortgages. The Century Convalescent chain, in which both Kosow and Geller were involved, approached the Forestville owners in 1970 with a proposal to lease the home and deposited, for this option, $135,000—an amount almost twice the value of the net assets of the home in 1970. The following year the management of Century and the owners of Forestville agreed to cancel the option; but Forestville returned only $45,000 of the deposit, while issuing a promissory note for the rest. In this deal between related parties who were seemingly unrelated, there is no explanation why the rest of the option money was not returned when the deal was called off. By the fall of 1971, Geller and his associates had reputedly sold the home to Walter Margerison, another Kosow associate. If that transaction ran true to form, the new owner would place a higher value on the home without changing its intrinsic worth, producing all the usual repercussions from that move.

It was the Connecticut Hospital Commission's belief that the estimated per-bed cost of $8,000 for nursing home construction could be reduced if the nursing home owner were to handle the contracting function personally. Material in the SEC files shows otherwise. Theoretically, by making economies in construction, a nursing home could turn those savings to improving care or raising wages and salaries. But just as government reimbursements help take the risk out of lending, so they remove the owners' instincts to economize, especially when the profits of a service, such as construction, go to the owners themselves. Economies in construction might mean a way to lower charges, a step seldom considered by owners; a rise in visible profits might weaken the case for higher reimbursements from government; improvements in care exceeding those reimbursed by government bring no added financial advantage; and excessively high salaries might well be questioned—if discovered. As a result, nursing home owners have an incentive to pay their affiliated companies more rather than less for services rendered, improving the earnings of these companies and avoiding embarrassing profits for the nursing homes.

One example of a home's failure to enjoy the advantages

accruing from its hold on other companies is to be found in SEC files on the Skyview Nursing Home—one of several Connecticut homes owned by a group of men including Guido Salvadore and Andrew Panteleakis of Rhode Island,

Skyview operated at a loss in 1970, perhaps because of the services rendered by companies owned by Panteleakis, alone or with Salvadore. A thirty-bed addition to Skyview was built by Panteleakis's construction company—at a cost exceeding the estimated cost of $8,000 per bed. Their equipment company sold the home its equipment at above-market prices, and Panteleakis's lending company held second and fourth mortgages on Skyview.

Meanwhile, the nursing home was accumulating a poor financial record. Every year since it opened in 1965 had ended with a declared loss (providing the partners with a useful tax loss to offset any profits elsewhere). The losses are not surprising in view of the prices charged by the owners' other companies for services to Skyview. Skyview is still operating, and its net worth in 1970, as reported to Connecticut authorities, exceeded that of 1969, as reported to the SEC. The question once again is, who will really bear the burden of excessive prices paid to related companies? Will the soup be watered, the staff cut, the linen not changed, soap and toilet paper disappear, and the government persuaded to pay more because the home appears to be losing money?

Back home in Cleveland, I witnessed a sequence of events in which a group of influential citizens bought a nursing home with great fanfare, then quickly and quietly dropped from sight. In February 1968 Cleveland newspapers heralded the purchase of Forest Hills, a 252-bed nursing home, by prominent Cleveland citizens. One was Frank Celeste, former mayor of Lakewood, a Cleveland suburb, and president of National Housing Consultants, a firm that produces housing for the elderly. Celeste introduced Sidney Spector as president of National Health Care Centers, a subsidiary company, and owner and operator of Forest Hills. Spector was a politically wise choice; he had been a consultant to Congress on housing for the elderly, and was soon to become a personal assistant to Mayor Carl Stokes of Cleveland.

I was invited to attend the gala opening of Forest Hills. Joy and hope filled that inaugural gathering. Dr. Joseph Molner, of Detroit, a syndicated columnist on health problems, spoke briefly. He told us he would commute between Detroit and Cleveland, a distance of 150 miles, to administer the home; he would continue to write his column; he was involved in a business designed to train nursing home personnel with customers as far away as California. It was a heady program of activities for one man, but no one seemed dismayed.

Mr. Spector was equally optimistic for his new corporation. He told the group, "I believe it is possible to provide a high-quality nursing home at a profit," catering to low- and middle-income families. The medical director for the home was introduced—Dr. Kenneth Clement, who had once served on a select sixteen-member commission for Social Security that wrote the standards for Medicare-approved homes, and who was then a special assistant to Mayor Stokes.

Newspapers published the names of the investors in Forest Hills; they were representatives of Cleveland wealth, political power, and the medical profession. Previously, they had merged their talents and money for other investment ventures extending into Europe and Soviet satellite countries. It was somewhat hard to understand why these international investors chose Forest Hills Nursing Home for their latest venture, especially since it would serve only persons of restricted income or those dependent on welfare.

So, with some fanfare, Forest Hills was launched. And almost immediately the clouds formed.

There is no evidence to show that the purported administrator, Dr. Molner, ever returned to Cleveland after delivering his speech on opening day. In any case, with no publicity, a successor to him was named. An interesting addendum to the story came within a month after the opening, when I visited Detroit. There I met a personal friend of Dr. Molner's and others who claimed to know him. None had heard of any connection between him and Forest Hills; none had heard of the school for training personnel to which he referred so glowingly on opening day. But one prominent person I met did say that he himself had been offered a similar chance to serve a nursing home in name only, without doing any work for his pay. Could this be the explanation for the mysterious Dr. Molner?

And the house kept tumbling down. Directors and investors listed by the newspapers were nowhere to be found in the names filed with the state health department within the year. Eight months after Sidney Spector had been named president of National Health Care Centers, Inc. {the corporation operating the home), neither his name nor the name of the corporation was listed as the operator or owner.

Almost from the beginning, negative reports on the kind of care offered at the home began to be heard from families and inspectors. In 1970 one elderly patient—a disabled man in his eighties—was charged with having bludgeoned his roommate to death. The old man was swiftly indicted for this crime, but as swift as that indictment was, it came after he had already been transferred to a mental institution on orders of Forest Hills's medical director, thus effectively discrediting him as a witness. The home's records describe this man who purportedly clubbed someone to death as unable to walk or dress himself without assistance, while the victim could do both. The supposed killer had never enjoyed the right to counsel, had no family, and was scarcely able to speak English. When, at last, the Legal Aid Society agreed to send a representative to see him at the mental institution, that representative emerged convinced that he was too frail to have murdered anyone. And among welfare officials, the story told was that an angry employee had actually been responsible for the fatal beating—a story that, if confirmed, would make the home liable to suit for extreme negligence.

A few weeks after that tragedy, the body of a patient was discovered on the flat roof of the home. The official version was that his death had been caused by a fall, evidenced by several broken ribs and severe bruises. It was determined that he had gone out on the roof and stumbled over one or more low dividers on its flat surface. Yet, according to the home's records, this man could neither walk nor climb stairs without assistance. According to the nurse's notes, his body was found four days after he was discovered to be missing, although the home and the roof had allegedly been searched at the time of his disappearance.

Finally, in the fall of 1971, a highly unfavorable report on the home was issued by a county welfare medical review team. But it caused neither public outrage nor changes in the home, since such reports are not brought to public attention. The team had found evidences of incorrect diagnoses, infrequent visits by the physician, no daily nursing notes, little cooperation between the dietary and nursing departments, drugs ordered by telephone without the required orders from a doctor, a shortage of linens, and patients being classified as needing maximum care when in fact they neither needed nor received such care.

What really happened at Forest Hills is unknown to me, because the information is not available. All the publicity about Forest Hills led one to believe that those prominent personalities were in fact the owners of the home. But the records of the state health department list only the operators, not the owners, and as noted earlier, all but one of the prominent names failed to appear on the state ownership form. There is no record of who owns the property itself: it may have been the same group, or it may have been still others. All that is certain is that the real owners, whoever they are, command enough influence around town to keep the home out of trouble with the regulating agencies.

These examples will, I hope, be enough to make the point: the abuses and rackets that pollute the nursing home industry will not be stopped until we find out who owns the industry. Government could do the job, if it wanted to. If I, one person alone, working from public records without official powers, could dig out the information given in this chapter, then government could easily uncover the whole pattern of ownership in the industry. All government needs is the will—and that is what is lacking.

Congress is the one arm of the federal government that has shown an occasional interest in finding out what is going on. Twice Congress has attempted to get information about nursing home ownership, and twice it has been defeated— the first time by the bureaucrats of HEW, the second by the states.

In 1967 Congress voted in the Moss Amendments (named for Senator Frank Moss of Utah, chairman of the Subcommittee on Long-Term Care), which required that ownership of Medicaid homes be revealed. This effort was quickly defanged by HEW, which interpreted the law to mean that only the ownership of companies operating (not necessarily owning) nursing homes needed to be revealed. This interpretation, which shielded real owners from the pain of disclosure, remains in effect. As to why HEW chose that route, see Chapter 10 for a description of the influence that nursing home representatives have exerted on that department.

The second effort came in 1970, when the Senate Finance Committee asked HEW to produce the names of all owners of Medicaid homes. HEW passed the request on to the states, which responded with mounds of non-information.

Here, for example, is how Connecticut answered the question (each being the complete statement on that home as submitted by the state):

> Keefe's Convalescent Hospital. Owner: Privately owned. Pineview Convalescent Hospital. Owner: Corporation. Thirty-Thirty Park Health Center. Owner: Church-sponsored.

Other states submitted equally empty replies. Michigan and Ohio agencies, for example, obeyed the requirement that names of corporate officers be revealed; but in what I saw, the requirement that principal stockholders be listed was ignored. Part of the Massachusetts response to the request that owners be named was the declaration that the Bigelow Nursing Home in Brighton, Massachusetts, is managed by the Bigelow Management Corporation. That tells us little enough—and besides it isn't even true. Actually, Bigelow is run by Eliot Management Company, a wholly owned subsidiary of Century Convalescent Homes. The fact that no one in state or federal agencies is assigned to check out ownership makes possible such contradictions.

That ended the second, and as of this writing, last effort to force federal and state bureaucracies to get the information on nursing home ownership. It is unlikely that any successful effort will be made in the near future, and it is still less likely that any effort will be made to reveal an even more secret group involved in the industry: the nursing home moneylenders.

6

The Moneylender: A More Secret Sharer

He is known, to those few who know both him and the industry, as "King of the Nursing Homes." To the press and the public at large, he is merely a "Boston financier," for his nursing home kingdom does not appear on the public record. Unlike Eugene Woods and Max Strauss, he does not have his name linked directly with the operation of nursing homes, and unlike Bernard Bergman, he does not make his money from owning them. Yet this reputed millionaire has himself declared nursing homes to be his chief source of income.

Joseph Kosow is a moneylender. He belongs to a category of profiteers whose activities in the nursing home industry are still more difficult to trace than the concealed owners. They do not show up in court, for there is nothing necessarily illegal about high interest rates, no matter what the effect may be on patient care. Only rarely has the baleful influence of the moneylender even been recognized. Once was by Allan Robinson, one-time counsel to a Massachusetts special commission that was studying nursing homes. Testifying in Boston before the Senate Subcommittee on Long-Term Care, Robinson spoke of "the loan .sharks who sat, and perhaps still sit astride many of the facilities, like fat spiders, and who have waxed rich on their shackled mortgagors."

Robinson, who identified Kosow as a "fat cat" who "has the nursing home industry in the palm of his hand," said a shoe-string operator could get started with Kosow's financing;

> They could walk in to Joe and literally buy a $100,000 home without putting down a nickel. Now what would one expect to be the outcome from that? . . . Of course he [Kosow] would write it on his terms, he would take the financing charges off the top and would have so much payable per week and at such a rate of interest. Before one got through he was paying in the thirties and around 40 percent [interest] at least. Compounded it would run considerably more than that perhaps.

Of moneylenders in general, Robinson said:

> I still see some of the fat spiders around, and, I am depressed to note, in the highest councils of the industry. At first they went underground, running real scared. Now they have emerged fatter, bolder and more cunning than ever.

That was in 1965. As far as I have been able to determine, Robinson's conclusion is just as sound today. Certainly Joseph Kosow is still around, unscathed by occasional investigation, his nursing home kingdom as strong and flourishing as ever. Still king in Massachusetts, he moved into Connecticut and most recently was reported operating in New York State.

The system Robinson was describing works through what are called lower-position mortgages, those that come after the traditional first mortgage. The first mortgage, familiar to homeowners, is given by a standard lending institution and carries an interest rate of between 5 and 8 percent. This is the safe mortgage, because if the property owner fails to make his payments and is foreclosed, the holder of the first mortgage gets first crack at his assets. Holders of second and third mortgages have to stand in line, and if there are no assets left after the first mortgage has been paid, they get nothing. Because they are riskier, lower-position mortgages naturally carry a higher—often much higher—rate of interest.

However, if the risk can be limited and the interest rate kept high, the lower mortgage can be extremely profitable. On $40,000, for example, a five-year mortgage at 40 percent (Robinson's figure) will earn $53,003; where a first mortgage at, say, 7 percent will bring in only $7,523. The trick is in limiting the risk. In the nursing home industry, of course, the risk of loss of income is virtually eliminated by guaranteed (and continually rising) government revenue. A second tactic is to place trusted associates as "owners" of the property to ensure that they will keep the mortgage payments coming in at the expense of all other considerations, including the welfare of the patients. The associate-owner can also collaborate to take out the mortgage with the lender and fix the interest as high as the traffic (i.e., the government) will bear, since the associate does not have the usual owner's motivation to keep the interest low. (He may also take out mortgages not needed for the nursing home.) Finally, if the burden of debt gets too heavy for government and patients jointly to shoulder, then a carefully staged foreclosure will get the lender and his associates out with a profit; an arranged bankruptcy will leave his associates virtually unscathed while other unwary creditors hold the bag.

That is what Kosow has done. As I will show in the cases described below, Kosow fastened on a group of nursing homes loans so large and at such high interest that over one-fourth of the income of those homes was used to meet the mortgage payments alone. During the frequent shuffling of "ownership" of the homes—they even belonged to a Texas bishop for a while—the one constant was the Kosow loans. Two of the listed owners went into bankruptcies that did not appear to hurt them much, if at all.*

* It should he remembered, in the descriptions of mortgage maneuvers in this chapter, that a nursing home owner who takes out a mortgage on his property is under no obligation to use the money to improve the home—

Government was, as usual, tolerant of these nursing home manipulations. When a Kosow associate wiped out his debts to the Federal Housing Administration by going into bankruptcy, the FHA responded by lending him some more money. Kosow himself was convicted of conspiracy to commit perjury during an SEC probe, but the conviction was reversed on appeal. Investigations of his activities came to nothing. Clear evidence of financial dealings between Kosow and the state official who regulated nursing homes was known to two successive attorneys general of Massachusetts, Edward M. Brooke and Elliot Richardson. They failed to act on the evidence, and have since gone on to higher things: one is a U.S. senator, the other, in April 1973, was named U.S. Attorney General after the Watergate scandal broke. A different reward was reserved for a state regulator who tried to do his job: when he was found to be immune to bribery, he was driven out of office.

The record of investigations and cases concerning Kosow, though incomplete and fragmentary, was enough to give me a start. Seeking to grasp how the money lending operator works, I spent weeks in Boston and Washington poring over documents and interviewing officials who knew something about Kosow. Those studies provided the information for the accounts that follow—accounts that, while complex and incomplete in places, Will provide a picture of how one person profited by money lending, at the public's expense, in the nursing home industry.

By way of introduction, here are some of the people and places involved:

Joseph Kosow owns and/or manages several investment

---

and therefore the care of patients. He can use the mortgage money to finance another business enterprise, or to buy a yacht, if he so chooses. Meanwhile his mortgage will be paid off by patient revenue, most of which comes from government. So the presence of second and third mortgages in no way indicates that the nursing home is not profitable. Indeed, the mortgage does not even prove that the money changed hands; its only purpose may be the payment of interest to the moneylender.

firms, some of them federally funded, that make loans to nursing homes. Has given conflicting versions of his role in the industry. Once told a court: "The major source of my income, sir, of my income, is from building and operating nursing homes, of which I am probably the largest in this state [Massachusetts] and that is where my particular income is derived from." Later told the Senate Subcommittee; "I own a lawful 50 percent interest in two nursing homes in Massachusetts. . . . My ownership of Massachusetts nursing homes amounts to one-third of one percent of the total of nursing homes in the Commonwealth." Net worth in the period described here rose from $2,590,000 to "$11 million plus." Used to drive a white Rolls Royce. Lives on Bald Pate Hill Road, in Newton, Massachusetts, as do his brother and a lawyer and contractor associated with him. Bald Pate Hill commands a lovely view, which is more than can be said for:

Neponset View Nursing Home, off Route 3 south of Boston. Despite the name, all one sees out the windows is the back side of a factory building. Patient prospects on a par with the view. Under burden of Kosow loans, debt per bed rose from $3,444 in 1958 to $8,469 in 1969. Was first of series of homes to get Kosow loans in association with:

Dr. *Frank C. Romano,* of Wellesley, Massachusetts, where he had a $97,000 Tudor house. Medical doctor, engaged since 1943 in buying and selling nursing homes. Served as owner of record for seven to nine homes carrying Kosow loans. Went into bankruptcy but bounced right back. Homes went on to:

Waldman and Carver. They make nonwoven labels, like the one for the convention circuit that says: "Hello! My name is ———." Their names appear as the officers of Geriatric Services, which takes over the group of homes, along with the Kosow loans, after Romano. They, too, go bankrupt without, however, appearing to be badly hurt by the action. Homes go on, with Kosow debt, to:

The Most Reverend L. J. Reicher, bishop of the Diocese of Austin, Texas. He holds homes three years, and manages apparently neither to win nor to lose on his venture. Homes, still with Kosow loans, go 011 to other ownership, leaving unaccounted for only:

Mac's Friendly Service Station, 1301 Blue Hill Avenue, Boston. This modest gas station is listed as the address of Geriatric Services and another corporation, businesses worth millions at one time. It was never explained why the corporations should choose to list themselves at a service station, even a friendly one.

Neponset View was the first nursing home involved in the manipulations we are about to trace. It will epitomize the effect that the moneylender has on nursing home costs—though it must be remembered that Kosow's operations were many times larger than what we are describing here, so the damage to the taxpayer, and to patient care, is correspondingly larger.

Romano acquired Neponset View with Kosow in 1958. Within about a year that home had been saddled with mortgages totaling $310,000, about twice the value of the home. The mortgages work out to $3,444 per bed, at a time when new construction, according to Kosow himself, cost around $1,400 per bed. The mortgages were held by Kosow, Romano himself and a third person. Romano also claimed that he bought out Kosow's share at some undisclosed later date, though this transaction is not apparent from the records.

Next, in 1959, Romano entered into a major borrowing deal with Kosow involving seven homes, one of them being Neponset. Romano mortgaged the homes to Kosow and associates for a loan with a face value of $1,292,084.67. Of this, $700,000 was the principal and $592,084.67 was interest added to the face value of the loan. It was to be repaid in 359 weekly installments of $3,600. The effective annual interest rate was 20 percent.

The loan, known as the Court Street Venture, had some

peculiar aspects besides the stiff interest rate. For one thing, not much of the money went to Romano himself. As the table below makes clear, a good part of the principal went to Kosow and his associates. Of the part listed as going to Romano, Kosow later testified that $157,000 went not to Romano but to Kosow.

Very little if any of the money went to the nursing homes themselves, to improve them or expand their capacity. Of the payments listed in Table i, the only one that could have been used for that purpose is the check to Dr. McCarty's Rest Home, and that is only $24,700—out of a total indebtedness of $1,200,000.

Table 1
PAYMENTS BY COURT STREET VENTURE NO. 1, JULY THROUGH OCTOBER 1959

Industrial Finance Corporation (Joseph Kosow's Company)	$109,666.54
Joseph Kosow	40,233.27
Joseph Buchhalter	139,219.00
Dr. McCarty's Rest Home	24,700.00
Frank C. Romano	104,025.00
Frank C. Romano	8,150.00
Frank C. Romano	5,000.00
Frank C. Romano	157,500.00
Frank C. Romano	7,500.00
Dr. Isreal Edelstein	40,200.00
Louis Bravo and Abraham K. Isenberg	25,500.00
Florence A and Amelia Crimmins	5,308.26
Julian H. Katzeff	27,500.00
Escrow	28.16

But the homes got the whole burden of meeting the $3,600 weekly payments, without any increase in their ability to pay. The annual income of the homes was between $750,000 and $850,000, according to a later court hearing:

let us put it at $800,000. Payments on the Court Street Venture loan totaled $187,200. Thus almost one-quarter of all patient revenue went to pay off this one loan (and there were also first mortgages on the homes). This was a heavy burden on the patients, whose care had to be scrimped so the loans could be paid. From the point of view of the taxpayer, a large slice of the money that supposedly was going to take care of patients was in fact being used to enrich Kosow and associates.

There was more and better to come. The next Kosow-Romano deal added to high interest the benefit of inflated construction costs (by this time, the per-bed debt at Neponset had been driven up to $8,424 from $3,444 a year earlier). This time Romano borrowed $141,000 from Kosow and associates to do some construction at one of the group of Romano homes, Dr. McCarty's. The interest on this loan, secured by all the Romano homes, was 15 percent. This seemed modest compared to the 20 percent charged by Kosow in the Court Street Venture, but this time the major profit came on the construction. Kosow was to do the construction. Romano paid him the $141,000 he had borrowed from him—and the construction actually cost Kosow $63,000. Thus Kosow recouped $206,292 (principal plus interest) on an outlay of $63,000; in other words, he more than tripled his money in five years (the term of the loan}, with the taxpayer, not Romano, picking up the bill via Medicaid. It is worth noting here that Romano must have known he could have gotten the loan at much lower interest from the Federal Housing Administration, since he had negotiated such loans for other nursing homes. Actually, this was one Kosow venture that may not have succeeded entirely. When Romano's bankruptcy was in court, the judge allowed $9,000 as a reasonable profit on the deal, and ordered Kosow to give back the rest (although I was unable to find any indication in the records that the restitution was actually made). Asked about his profit, Kosow replied: "When I quote a price on the job, I don't go around telling people what I make on it, sir." He explained that the profit had not gone to him at all, but to "the Sherman-Kosow Family Venture" (Isadore Sherman was an associate of Kosow).

Kosow described how he had protected his loan, indicating his effective ownership of the homes. He appointed one of his own lawyers, Arthur Wasserman (his neighbor on Bald Pate Hill, as well as an investor in the Court Street Venture) as an officer of the homes to represent the lender. Kosow made this appointment, he explained, so "Dr. Romano would not go into extra heavy dealing with some of his former friends or business acquaintances at rates that make me look like a Lord Fauntleroy."

Kosow also assigned two individuals to operate the seven homes belonging to Dr. Romano. One was the certified public accountant who testified that he was unaware of the fact that the money from the Sherman-Kosow loan, secured by the seven homes, had actually been used for improvements to only one home. The accountant also admitted that he was not really sure what his relationship to the corporation was—whether he was a director or simply the accountant.

The other man chosen by Kosow to operate the homes was Arthur Blasberg, Jr., an attorney hired from the Securities and Exchange Commission in Washington. This is the Arthur Blasberg, Jr., who is now chairman of the executive committee of the board of directors of Health Care Corporation, to one of whose homes in New Hampshire President Nixon, in search of a model nursing home, was directed.

The Sherman-Kosow loan added only $333 to the per-bed debt at Neponset (which was part of the collateral for that loan). This brought the per-bed debt up to $8,757 or six times what it cost Kosow to put in beds under the Sherman-Kosow loan.

By now, the Kosow loans were siphoning off more than half the assumed profits on the seven homes held in Romano's name. At the bankruptcy hearing, Romano said there were 400 beds in the seven homes, and Kosow himself commented that: "It was felt that a nursing home could average a net operating profit before debt of approximately $1,000 a year per bed—before interest and principal on the mortgage." This means the Romano homes should have been netting about $400,000 a year. Of this, the Kosow loans were eating up $230,676 for the Court Street and Sherman-Kosow loans.

Note in passing that Kosow was confirming what the industry always denies except when it is selling shares— that it is an extremely profitable business. If, as Kosow said, an operator can make a net operating profit of $1,000 per bed, and if the cost of the new construction Kosow did for Romano works out to $1,400, that means an annual return of 71 percent on the investment. You can pay a lot to the moneylender on that kind of return.

Things looked pretty good for the Kosow interests, but for reasons that do not appear in the record, it was evidently not good enough. The next round of maneuvers over Neponset and the other six homes culminated in the declaration of bankruptcy by Dr. Romano. Before that happened, however, and this was crucial to the maneuver, the homes had been taken out of his name by a series of manipulations to be described below. When Romano went into bankruptcy, the general interpretation was that he had been exploited by Kosow. According to most observers, the moneylender had pushed Romano, the innocent nursing home operator, against the wall by saddling him with debts, then had tossed him aside when he could not meet the payments.

In my opinion, this official version does not stand the test of logic. In fact, Romano does not seem to have suffered at all from his bankruptcy (while Kosow, as we shall see, benefited). The effect of the bankruptcy proceedings was to wipe out Romano's debts, but this had no effect on Kosow, whose loans had gone along with the homes when they were taken out of Romano's name. When his assets were added up, the sum was $11,915. No one got anything except Internal Revenue, which collected $8,000 on hack taxes of $32,000. The rest of the $11,915 went to the lawyers.

Government once again appears as the eternal sucker. Among Romano's debts wiped out by the bankruptcy was $7,240 he owed the Federal Housing Administration. He had borrowed in 1960 and again in 1961 under the FHA's program providing loans for nursing home improvements, and he had not paid his debt off by the time he went bankrupt in October 1962. Now the FHA was out the whole amount. But this past history deterred neither Romano nor the agency.

In 1963, Romano's son and son-in-law organized as Holyoke Nursing Home, giving Romano's home as their address. In 1965 the name of the corporation is changed to R & R Nursing Home; the names of the directors are also changed. The purpose of the corporation, according to the articles of organization, was "to get FHA financing." And get it they did. In 1967 Dr. Romano turns up as operator of what is again called the Holyoke Nursing Home, on which the FHA has insured a mortgage for $845,700. In the spring of 1971 I attempted to find why FHA would have backed Romano for still another loan, but a conversation with FHA officials in Washington resulted only in the promise that I could get the information from their regional office. I was told in passing that applicants for loans are required to fill out a form, 2530, which lists their previous dealings with the FHA. When I telephoned the regional office, I was told that Romano was indeed listed as the owner of Holyoke Nursing Home and that it had received the loan. When I asked why they had given him the loan in view of his history, I was told that all applicants are investigated. For further information, I was told, write the regional director, Daniel Richardson. I did so. As of this writing, two years later, I still await his reply.

There is another way of looking at this episode. The loan was applied for under a name other than Romano's,

134 · Tender Loving Greed

with the doctor emerging after the transaction was complete. (The application was made by Fontain Brothers, a construction company that was later bought by a nursing home chain, Geri-Care, that was linked to the Kosow interests.) Yet the point remains the same: government lets itself be had. If the intent of the FHA rules can be as easily evaded as it was in this case, then those rules have no meaning, and FHA officials must be aware of that fact. In any event, this is how the transactions between Romano and the government add up. He owed a total of $39,240 ($7,240 to the FHA and $32,000 to Internal Revenue); government collected $8,000 of that amount, then insured a loan for his operation of another $845,700.

Dr. Romano now leaves our story, after one final action. In November 1961 Romano defaulted on his payments on the two Kosow loans. This permitted the Kosow interests to foreclose on the loans and transfer ownership of the seven nursing homes before Romano went into bankruptcy. The homes and loans went on to another set of owners: Waldman and Carver of the Waldoroth Label Company and a new corporation called Geriatric Services. Interestingly enough, Geriatric Services was the successor to a corporation, Nursing Homes, Inc., which Waldman and Carver had formed with Kosow associates as far back as 1958—before the Romano foreclosure and even before the Court Street Venture loan. The switch of the nursing homes to this supposedly new group was accomplished by a series of maneuvers of which George Broomfield, receiver in the Romano bankruptcy, testified:

> Kosow, acting with other defendants [which included Geriatric Services] did conspire and agree to gain possession and control of the Receivership Corporation [Neponset View] and other similar corporations [the other six nursing homes] by a scheme to have all the Corporations sign a joint and several note in the sum of $1,292,084.67, which

far exceeded any single corporation asset . . . and further, by causing Wasserman to become Clerk of the various Corporations . . . and then causing a series of fraudulent mortgages, including the $30,000 mortgage [Neponset View's share of the Sherman-Kosow loan] to be executed and then foreclosed, with their agreement to control the sales. . . . the sales were tainted with fraud, were controlled, the indebtednesses were overstated, the property sold for grossly inadequate prices, and were contrary to equity and fair dealing.

As has been mentioned, Kosow bad assigned a certified accountant and a lawyer to manage the Romano homes for a time. When Dr. Romano discontinued his weekly payments on his mortgage loans, this sequence of events followed, engineered largely through Barney Goldstein, a foreman at the Waldoroth Label Company (only Neponset View is used here as an example, though the other six homes owned by Romano were also involved in the transactions):

1. *November 25, 1961:* The Court Street Venture group assigned its loan in the original amount of $1,292,084.67 to Barney Goldstein.

2. *November 25, 1961:* The Sherman-Kosow loan to Dr. Romano (Neponset's share was $30,000) was assigned to another Kosow finance company, Congress Management Corporation.

3. *November 25, 1961:* Congress Management assigned the Sherman-Kosow loan to Court Street Venture.

4. *November 25, 1961:* Court Street Venture assigned the Sherman-Kosow loan to Barney Goldstein for $991,661.

5. *November* 25, 1961; Barney Goldstein was named the trustee of a trust for the benefit of Waldman, Wallins, and Carver. (Wallins had recently joined the other two in their nursing home venture.) Address—1301 Blue Hill Avenue. That's Mac's Friendly Service Station.

6. *March 29, 1962:* Neponset View sold by foreclosure.

Purchaser—Barney Goldstein. Price—$2,500, subject to a first mortgage and a second mortgage to secure $1,292,-084.67 (the Court Street Venture).

7. *March 30, 1962;* Another sale by foreclosure of the same property is recorded, subject to first mortgage. Purchaser—Barney Goldstein. Price—$35,000.

8. *April 30, 1962;* Mortgage from Barney Goldstein to Court Street Venture and Industrial Small Business Investment Corporation (Kosow's) to secure payment of notes of November 25,1961.

(And then, days later, a new name enters the land deed record: Geriatric Services, Inc.)

9. *May 9, 1962:* Deed from Barney Goldstein, Trustee, to Geriatric Services, consideration $35,000, subject to first and second mortgages.

10. *July 2, 1962:* Mortgage from Geriatric Services to Congress Management Corporation, $160,000, subject to a first mortgage of $125,000 (held by Dr. Israel Edelstein) and second mortgage of Barney Goldstein, Trustee, to Court Street Venture in the approximate sum of $929,661.00.

The whole weird sequence of transfers of deeds, assignments, and mortgage arrangements was a means of transferring the Romano homes, complete with their mortgages, to a new group of owners with a surface appearance of arm's-length agreements. Barney Goldstein, the intermediary, dropped from sight. Along with the homes, the new owners acquired the obligation to pay off the indebtedness owed to Kosow's lending companies. The corporation's officers then gave still another mortgage to another lending company dominated by Kosow. Thus Kosow seemed to have improved his position considerably. There was only one substantial cash payment, $35,000, made for the purchase of Neponset. Still, some money from some deal, perhaps the Court Street Venture loan, paid off the mortgage notes given earlier to Romano, Kosow, and Sherman-Kosow. The Court Street

Venture loan, with its egregious interest payments, was carried over, and Kosow had fastened another mortgage, for $160,000, on Neponset. His mortgages now totaled $1,214,-661.

By now, despite payments on earlier mortgages over the years, the debt per bed at poor old Neponset—and the building, unimproved, was not getting any younger—was $5,490, about four times the replacement cost.

The new owner, Geriatric Services, was the creation of Jacob Waldman and Joseph Carver, the label manufacturers. They had dabbled in enterprises other than labels before they created Geriatric Services, and some of these earlier ventures had mirrored Kosow's modes of operation. Waldman and Carver, too, were moneylenders, with some loans going to liquor interests and a second mortgage advanced to at least one of their own nursing homes, a facility held by a Kosow nominee. Details of their various ventures are almost impossible to trace. How many loans their lending companies have advanced to nursing homes, by what means they entered the business as owners and lenders, are facts I could not uncover. What is known is that Joseph Carver and Jacob Waldman appeared on the nursing home scene in 1958, in the period when so many others entered the business; and they arrived connected with Charles Brennick, who was, and is, allied with Joseph Kosow. Brennick and his brothers hold the deeds to many homes on which they have placed lower-position mortgages with Kosow's lending companies. From time to time, those homes have been deeded from the Brennicks to Walter Margerison (a Brennick brother-in-law) or to James Martin, both Kosow associates. Along with Margerison and Martin, the Brennicks today are the deed holders of nursing homes being moved into public chains, carrying with them, in the transfers, the mortgages held by Kosow.

The Waldman-Carver involvement in nursing homes expanded rapidly. By 1961 they were ready to go to the public for additional capital through an offering of stock. (The date shows that they were pioneers in the art of adding stockholders to the patients and the taxpayers as victims of nursing home hustles. See the following chapter for more on this aspect of the business.) Geriatric Services, organized in 1960, circulated its prospectus encouraging prospective stock purchasers in the fall of 1961. The company burst forth with fourteen homes and promises of a glorious future. That bright future would see the retirement of some debts, with an estimated 50 percent of the proceeds to go to the modernization and expansion of the homes. They sought to raise $300,000 from investors. (A third man, Paul Wallins, had joined Waldman and Carver by this time.)

The public records concerning Geriatric Services contain several inaccuracies. Even the addresses given for some of the nursing homes are inaccurate. Indeed, one of the more curious mistakes, the meaning of which can only be surmised, is the fictitious address of the company. That address, as filed with the Massachusetts secretary of state, on mortgage records, and in general references, is 1301 Blue Hill Avenue. During these same years, 1301 Blue Hill Avenue is listed in the city directories as the address variously of the Lipson Oil Company, Mac's Friendly Service Station, Bob and Fred Service Station, until finally the address disappears from the directory. Nor is the listing of the company at that address accidental, since Geriatric Services was also listed in the telephone book with a number at the gas station. (Another corporation involved in managing these same homes was later to use Mac's as its address.) A different address was given in the Geriatric Services prospectus—1261-1295 Blue Hill Avenue, but the prospectus does not reveal that this address is that of Carver and Waldman's Waldoroth Label Company. When the correct address appears in the prospectus, and occasionally elsewhere, the theory that a clerk might have typed a wrong number that was then copied by all other clerks is not a satisfactory answer. When a telephone in the company's name is installed at the gasoline station address, the error ceases to be error and becomes obvious subterfuge. But why hide their business address? It is one of the more fascinating mysteries in the nursing home business. (This practice of listing false addresses can be found in other nursing home operations. For example, in late 1971 the officers of a large, public California-based chain were found to be using wrong addresses, even listing a vacant lot for one corporation they owned. The reason in that case for the dummy address was that the corporation never existed.)

In addition to its inaccuracies, the prospectus revealed some seldom-seen details of the budgets of the acquired nursing homes. These details illustrate the effect of mortgage deals. One home, the Crawford Nursing Home, serves as the prototype of many. Crawford was an aging home, described as brick-front and stucco-frame construction, licensed for forty-nine patients. There were, of course, the inevitable mortgages. The first mortgage was with the City Bank and Trust Company, whose president was Kosow's associate in a number of transactions; and a second mortgage was assigned to Central Acceptance Plan, a lending company controlled by Waldman and Carver, and located at the Waldoroth Company address. In 1959 these mortgages totaled $127,000—an inflated amount of $2,600 per bed, compared to Kosow's own cost for new construction of $1,400 per bed. Buried in the prospectus was an ironic note on the value of the Crawford Home. Because of the condition of the records kept by the predecessors, the prospectus stated, the valuation could not be given to the public in the financial statement.

This was strange, since, as we have seen, Crawford two years earlier had secured a mortgage held by the Central Acceptance Plan, Waldman and Carver's firm. The officers of Crawford at that time included Waldman and Carver. Waldman and Carver, we are asked to believe, as the officers of the Central Acceptance Plan and officers of the nursing home that obtained the mortgage, could not ascertain the value of the property they owned (on one side) and for which they risked their company's money (on the other side). Waldman and Carver, now as officers of Geriatric Services, had apparently kept their secret from themselves.

The income and expense figures for Crawford, attached to the prospectus, clearly reveal what inflated mortgages do to the patient-care budget. Rent (including the mortgage payments) ate up almost one-third of all revenue. Payroll costs, which normally take close to two-thirds of revenue, took only one-third. The remaining one-third had to pay for all the rest: food, supplies, linen, maintenance, heat, utilities. And the per-bed debt was to get still higher for all the homes after the next transaction involving them.

Geriatric Services also introduced the currently popular practice of centralizing various administrative functions, such as bookkeeping and consultant services. Normally, the idea is to cut the costs of operating individual homes, but that was not the idea at Geriatric. Geriatric Services, the parent company, sold these services to Crawford at an inflated cost: they charged Crawford almost as much for bookkeeping services as Crawford spent for food. Or, to put it the other way around, Crawford spent as little for food as it did for bookkeeping. It takes no imagination to realize that Crawford could not, and did not, serve three nutritious meals a day to each patient; or that Crawford did not have adequate numbers of trained staff members. Geriatric Services' profits were being shifted out, and the patients were paying off the mortgages.

Geriatric Services sold $300,000 in common stock to the public in October 1961, with the promoters keeping the preferred stock. In line with the pledges in the prospectus as to how the proceeds would be spent, the next steps should have been the modernization of the homes Geriatric already owned and the retirement of debt. Instead, most of that money went to buying the seven Romano homes at the staged foreclosure.

Within a few months, Geriatric Services owned a total of twenty-three nursing homes—a respectable collection, if not yet an empire. It didn't last long. Within a year, in mid-1963, Geriatric had sold their homes to, of all people, the Roman Catholic bishop of Austin, Texas, the Most Reverend L. J. Reicher.

The deal was arranged by a new promoter on the scene. Howard Lawn had graduated *summa cum laude* from Harvard College, then from Harvard Law School. After a brief stint as assistant U.S. attorney in New Jersey, he became an executive of American Brands Corporation, and that is where he got into trouble. He was convicted on a corporate tax evasion charge and served five months of a one-year sentence; during the trial, it came out that a co-defendant and officer of the firm also worked as an accountant for Joe Profaci, the late don of a Brooklyn Mafia family. Lawn later appeared as an agent for Clove Lakes Realty Corporation, the landholding company of the Austin Diocese. It was from this vantage point that Lawn swung the deal for the nursing homes.

Waldman and Carver, the promoters of Geriatric Services, were later to tell Senate investigators that they were forced to sell because of the high interest they were paying to Kosow. Geriatrics had mortgages on its homes totaling nearly $3,600,000, most of it owed to Kosow and his associates. Kosow, they said, was charging them up to 3 percent a month on their loans, and they were having trouble meeting their bills. What the enterprise needed, they concluded, was "respectable" financing, and who could better obtain respectable financing than a bishop? Since Waldman and Carver, as well as Kosow, profited from the sale to the bishop, there is considerable room for doubt in their explanation. Still, the deal was made, the Boston *Traveler* calling it "the largest of its type in the Bay State." These were the transactions as the twenty-three nursing homes moved into "respectable" financing:

1. The respected Boston Five Cents Savings Bank (a commercial bank) entered the ranks of those willing to lend money to nursing homes. In a refinancing action, the bank advanced $2.8 million, acquiring a first mortgage position on the twenty-three nursing homes.

2. The Industrial Finance Corporation (a Kosow company that had been sold to Merrit-Chapman Scott but was still managed by Kosow) took a second mortgage position for $800,000.

3. Geriatric Services was given a non-interest-bearing promissory note for $4.7 million. The common stock of the corporation had grown to a paper worth of almost $5 million —now the principal asset of the company.

4. Jacob Waldman, Paul Wallins, and Joseph Carver, holders of 78 percent of the preferred stock of the corporation, received $350,000 for that stock, the only preferred stock redeemed. This was the only major amount of cash involved in the sale of the twenty-three homes. (The holders of common stock got no cash.)

The bishop's Clove Lakes Realty Corporation had acquired along with the nursing homes an indebtedness that had more than doubled. The $3.6 million debt, which the former owners had given as their reason for selling, now stood at $8.3 million. The Boston Five Cents Savings Bank mortgage had paid off the old mortgage debt, owed primarily to Kosow's firm. Kosow, however, remained in the picture with his second mortgage. Waldman, Wallins, and Carver, alone of the stockholders, had gotten back a large share of their investment in Geriatric Services; the common stockholders had been assured that they, too, would profit by the move. They did not. In fact, their stock became worthless.

Howard Lawn was to operate the homes. Rather than send a management team out from Texas, Bishop Reicher immediately leased all the properties back to Geriatric Management, Lawn's company (which also gave as its address Mac's Friendly Service Station). Lawn then negotiated an eight-year contract with the trio of former owners, under which they were to be paid $50,000 annually for their work as operators while they continued to run their principal businesses (for Waldman and Carver, their label company). Experienced management would, the contract implied, produce savings for the homes and improved care for the patients.

The arrangement was incredible. The nursing homes, under those same operators, had skirted financial disaster, avoided only by the refinancing through the bank. After that refinancing, further debts were added, with some of the loans coming from the same source, Kosow, that had, the previous owners said, created the need for refinancing.

Nonetheless, everyone had done well out of the deal. Kosow had about $2 million of his earlier loans paid off by the bank, while keeping $800,000 in second mortgages— presumably at his usual high rates—on the homes. Howard Lawn collected a salary, and was even able to make a loan of $80,000 to another firm of his from the nursing home operation. Waldman, Wallins, and Carver got back their own investment in Geriatric preferred stock and collected their management salary on their eight-year contract. (Later they, like Romano before them, were to go through a bankruptcy proceeding that wiped out their debts but not their businesses.) The only losers were, as usual, the taxpayers forced to pay higher rates for the Kosow loans and the nursing home patients squeezed by the same loans—joined this time by those persons unwary enough to have invested in Geriatric Services common stock.

An ironic sidelight on the bishop's participation in the deal was provided in a 1964 report, catalogued by the Federal Reserve Bank of Boston, on "financing nursing homes." The study, by George E. Wells, advises banks to go into nursing

homes as a "sound and profitable enterprise," adding the
thought that if the home takes welfare patients this acts as
a "built-in stabilizer" of its income, since such homes have
close to 100 percent occupancy rates. Then the study cites
the bishop to prove its point;

> The nursing home as a sound business enterprise was well
> demonstrated recently by the purchase for investment pur-
> poses only of 22 Massachusetts homes for approximately
> $4.7 million by the Roman Catholic Diocese of Austin, Tex-
> as. It is anticipated that the earnings of these homes over
> the next 15 years will aggregate the $4.7 million purchase
> price.

It's reassuring to learn that even the Federal Reserve
Bank is not omniscient. What it did not know was that the
earnings of the homes would be drained off to pay oft the
burden of the Kosow loans and other debts,

In any event, the arrangement did not last nearly the
fifteen years mentioned by the Federal Reserve Bank. Only
three years later, in the summer of 1966, the holders of the
mortgages moved in to foreclose on the bishop's Clove
Lakes Realty Corporation. The Boston Five Cents Savings
Bank brought the first foreclosure action to recoup its 1964
loan of $2.8 million. Joseph Kosow moved next, demanding
payment for his second-position mortgage loan of $800,000.
Geriatric Services, holding its third-position $4.7 million
promissory note, did nothing. The old Romano-Geriatric
Services homes were sold at auction.

Kosow made out exceedingly well in this auction: the
record is clearer here than in some of the earlier transactions. The procedure at such a sale is for the holder of the
first mortgage (the bank) to auction enough homes to satisfy its debt, then the holder of the second mortgage (Kosow) auctions off what remains. During the first auction,
the Kosow interests bought four homes for $1,185,000, re-

sold them for $1,223,000, and placed mortgages on them for $1,395,000. In the second auction, the Kosow interests bought eight homes for $504,500, sold them for $753,300, and placed new mortgages for $380,000. Kosow had started out the transaction with $800,000 in mortgages. He ended it with a profit on the sales of $286,000 and mortgages totaling $1,775,000. It had been a good day's work.

The smooth cooperation between Kosow, holder of the second mortgage, and the holder of the first mortgage, the Boston Five Cents Savings Bank, was not surprising, since the bank had hired to advise it in the foreclosure a man who had done business with Kosow in the past. Richard Gens was still another hustler entering a situation that was already well supplied with that breed. He was well connected politically, having been an assistant attorney general of Massachusetts. He had interests in a number of nursing homes, though just how many I could not establish for sure, since Gens, like Bernard Bergman, set up separate corporations for each of his operations. In at least one nursing home deal, he did business with Abraham Gosman, a Kosow associate.* (One of Gosman's homes, by the way, was used as collateral for a loan to finance a movie called *Which Way Do You Dig?*) Another home, in which both Gens and Kosow had been involved, received a third mortgage from the First Connecticut Small Business Investment Corporation, a principal stockholder in Bernard Bergman's Medic-Homes chain. Thus at last there appeared in the public record what Senate investigators had long tried to establish: a connection between the interests of Joseph Kosow and those of Bernard Bergman. It is these kinds of connections, almost entirely buried from public view, that lead some of us to believe that power in the nursing home industry, apparently scattered

---

*On May 11, 1973, Richard Gens was found guilty on eleven counts of misappropriating bank funds insured by the FDIC. He was sentenced to prison for three years, and fined $10,000.

among many small owners, is in fact concentrated in relatively few hands, and that they are the hands of people like
Bernard Bergman and Joseph Kosow.

Neponset View, the home we have used to illustrate the
effect on costs of the moneylender, remained with Kosow
after it left the bishop's fold. It was sold to two Kosow associates, who resold it to still another, Dr. David Levy, who
at last reports still held it, its name having been changed in
1972 to Hilltop Manor. The home had been in Kosow hands
since 1958, and by 1969 this is what had happened to it: the
mortgages had risen from $310,000 in 1958 to $762,000 in
early 1969; the cost per bed of the mortgages had risen from
$3,444 to $8,469 a decade later.

That is only one of the many homes carrying Kosow
loans, and Kosow himself is only one of the moneylenders operating in the nursing home industry. Indeed, there
is evidence that his methods are widely practiced in the industry. The promoters of the nursing home chains described
in the next chapter frequently have their own finance companies, companies that give lower-position mortgages (not
first mortgages) on the homes. When the chain sells stock
to the public, one of the promises to the investor is that his
money will be used to pay off those mortgages. In the cases
I have examined, however, the mortgages were not in fact
paid off, doubtless because they were too profitable for the
promoters. Dr. Bernard Bergman, whom we met in the last
chapter, is one chain promoter who also has a finance company. There is in fact a natural connection between the excessive leases of a Bergman-style operation and the excessive interest of a Kosow mortgage, since both serve as ways
to drain profits out of the nursing home while driving up
the rate charged to the government. The cost to the taxpayer
of this kind of moneylending is unknown—because nursing
home regulators have made no attempt to find out—but it is
my belief that the bill, if we could ever calculate it, would
prove to be enormous. For the moneylender, there is the

great advantage that what he is doing is legal, no matter what it costs the rest of us.

The cost is likely to go up if the operators have their way on an issue that was agitating the industry early in 1973. The federal government was urging states that paid for Medicaid patients on a flat-rate basis to shift to a formula that would reimburse the operators for their costs, with the profit to be calculated on their equity in the home—which is essentially how Medicare now functions. The theory was that the change in payment systems would eliminate the incentive for the operator to increase profits by cutting his spending on patient care. The owners resisted the change. In Ohio, one state where the issue was raised, the owners argued that if the change was made their profit should be figured on the total capital asset value of the nursing home, not just on their equity in it. This, of course, would provide a bonanza for owner and moneylender alike. They could load as many high-interest mortgages on the homes as they liked (and use the proceeds for any purpose they chose), secure in the knowledge that the government would pay the extra cost and that their profits would be calculated on a value artificially inflated by those very mortgages.

The industry from which Kosow has made his fortune is largely financed by government, and, in theory at least, regulated by government. Kosow's career, like that of others in the business, is therefore dependent on the goodwill of government—goodwill expressed sometimes by active cooperation, at others by simply looking the other way. There is evidence that Kosow has enjoyed both kinds of goodwill. He has been in and out of the courts, but never seriously harmed. In one case, that of the Sherman-Kosow loan, he was ordered to give back his excess profits, but that was only one among Kosow's many deals. He has been investigated by the SEC and the Senate Subcommittee on Long-Term Care, but the evidence turned up in those investigations has never led to any conclusive action.

One form of government cooperation with Kosow was revealed in the record of Dr. Romano's bankruptcy. Testimony in that case was as follows:

The commissioner of welfare promised Romano that he would see to it that all their nursing home beds would be kept full with Medicaid patients; Kosow testified to his knowledge of Romano's good connections with welfare; the Board of Building Appeals allowed Kosow to use cheaper than required building materials for the construction he did for Romano; the Zoning Board allowed Kosow to squeeze in more than the permitted number of beds. All these exemptions increased Kosow's profit on the Sherman-Kosow transaction.

A more serious case was that of the financial dealings between Kosow and the state's chief nursing home regulator. This information also grew out of a court case. This time it was a suit for slander, brought against Joseph Kosow by Paul Wallins of Geriatric Services. Ultimately Wallins's case was dismissed with prejudice and with no right of appeal.

The most important information in the case had nothing to do with Wallins's suit, nor did it emerge from the courtroom. Rather, it was in a deposition taken in connection with the suit, a portion of which was leaked to the press. Records of depositions are not always easy to come by. They need not be filed with the court; the notice that they have been taken is registered on the court docket where the numbers and dates of depositions in connection with a case are listed. Thus the docket of the U.S. District Court revealed that depositions had been received from Paul Wallins., Joseph Kosow, the New England Merchants National Bank, and A. Daniel Rubenstein, M.D., the director until 1970 of the Massachusetts Division of Hospital Facilities, under whose aegis was the nursing home licensing division. The fragments of the Wallins deposition recalled the time in 1961 when he, Joseph Carver, and Jacob Waldman were about to acquire the nursing homes then owned by Dr. Romano.

Since these homes carried the burden of the Court Street Venture and Sherman-Kosow loans, the income from them had effectively been preassigned. The new owners could not afford to divert that income toward correcting health and safety violations. Hence, the attitude of the state health department toward the enforcement of its regulations was a critical factor.

It was then the policy of the Massachusetts Division of Hospital Facilities that, when more than 50 percent of the stock of a nursing home changed hands, the home would have to be brought into line with the latest regulations. This policy was a source of worry to Wallins. As he explained in the deposition, "One of the major concerns that Mr. Waldman and Mr. Carver and I expressed in purchasing those seven homes was the possibility that when the homes would change ownership, that we would have to conduct substantial repairs on those nursing homes." To conform to the official policy, he noted, might have meant cutting down on the number of beds.

Wallins then recalled a meeting in Joseph Kosow's office at which his worries were eased. As he put it in the deposition, "Mr. Kosow said to us, 'Don't worry about that. I can handle that part of it.' And I said that we were very much concerned, because even with refinancing, this could involve a substantial amount of money and we would be in trouble. So Mr. Kosow said, 'Well, if you want to be sure that you will not be bothered, meet me in my house on Sunday morning/ And the following Sunday morning at about nine o'clock I arrived at Mr. Kosow's house with Mr. Carver, Mr. Waldman, and a Dr. Rubenstein."

The counsel asked, "This is Dr. Daniel Rubenstein, is it not?"

"Yes," said Wallins.

"Do you recall what his official position was?"

"Dr. Rubenstein was head of all hospitals and nursing homes in the Commonwealth of Massachusetts."

Wallins continued: "Mr. Kosow told Dr. Rubenstein that Mr. Kosow was negotiating with us for the acquisition of seven Romano homes, and Mr. Kosow told Dr. Rubenstein that we were deeply concerned about having to spend considerable sums of money if it was necessary for us to make substantial repairs and bring the homes up to the latest requirements, which could be necessary when a nursing home changes ownership.

"Mr. Kosow said to Dr. Rubenstein, 'I want you to leave these fellows alone for at least one year.'

"Dr. Rubenstein said to Mr. Kosow, 'Okay, Joe, if that is the way you want it, it is all right with me.'"

Good reason for it to be "all right" with Dr. Rubenstein came out in a further investigation by the SEC. Its investigators turned up three checks, totaling $33,000, made out to Dr. Rubenstein and issued at around the same time as the Sunday morning meeting described by Paul Wallins. The checks—voucher-type checks on whose face the purpose for which the check was written was stated—were drawn on Kosow's account at the New England Merchants Bank. One of those checks acknowledged payment by Kosow to Dr. Rubenstein for his investments in a Kosow real estate operation called the Florida Deal. It was also discovered that Rubenstein had a financial interest in, and was a director of, one of Kosow's Small Business Investment corporations.

The fragment of Wallins's deposition and the checks to Dr. Rubenstein were, in 1966, given to the Senate Subcommittee on Long-Term Care. The subcommittee turned over the evidence to the then attorney general of Massachusetts, Edward M. Brooke, along with an offer of more evidence. A year earlier, after the subcommittee's hearings in Boston, the attorney general had declared that he was investigating alleged malpractices in the industry.

Upon receipt of the fresh evidence, Attorney General Brooke responded promptly, with thanks for the subcommittee's deferral of any action on its part until a full evaluation could be made of his own findings. He admitted the relevance of the Rubenstein transactions to his own investigation, but ignored the subcommittee's offer to make available to him the considerable additional information it had collected on the subject. Brooke's letter closed with the assurance that he would be glad to furnish the results of his .investigation to the subcommittee. This, however, he was never to do; nor did he tell the subcommittee the exact nature of his investigations, nor name individuals and homes being investigated.

Having heard nothing from Brooke between March and November 1966, the subcommittee again wrote the attorney general (just elected United States senator, but at the time still attorney general), asking for information on the results of the investigation. His complete reply on the subject, dated several weeks later, was:

> Our investigation has been thorough, and many facts relating to these matters have been collected. To date, some evidence has been developed of irregular and questionable actions, and corrective actions appear to have been taken within the Department concerned. I am not in possession of sufficient probative facts at this time to state that these irregular and questionable actions were of a criminal nature.
>
> The investigation is continuing. You undoubtedly have been informed concerning the considerable litigation which is underway involving many of the individuals who were concerned with the nursing home operations, which are the subject of this investigation. This had directly affected our success in obtaining any possible probative facts, which might otherwise have been obtained.

That letter closed the correspondence between the Senate subcommittee and the attorney general regarding Joseph Kosow and Dr. A. Daniel Rubenstein. It is noteworthy that Brooke's letter contained neither those names nor any others: no matter who saw it, the letter would not hurt anyone in the nursing home business.

Brooke's earlier investigation had to do with the attempted bribery of the director of licensing by nursing home owners. The allegation of attempted bribery was made by Dr. Samuel Levey, then administrator of nursing homes and related services in the Massachusetts Health Department., before the Senate subcommittee hearing in Boston. (Rubenstein, though still in the health department, was no longer in charge of licensing nursing homes.) Replying to a question by Senator Frank Moss as to whether he had been tendered bribes or favors, Dr. Levey said, "There have been attempts by the nursing home people to assist me in taking trips and acquiring various material things." In an interview with a reporter, he later added that he had advised the attorney general's office of these offers.

There followed a confusing dialogue among officials. A spokesman for the attorney general denied that an official complaint of attempted bribery had been made by the nursing home division. Then the health commissioner declared that he himself had given the information to an assistant attorney general, upon which the attorney general came forth in person to declare that he had already launched "an investigation into charges of criminal activity in the nursing home field." He claimed his office had information beyond that given by Dr. Levey to the subcommittee, and he hinted that his investigation had been going on for some time.

That investigation was buried with the attorney general's uninformative letter to the Senate subcommittee. As for Kosow's relationships with Rubenstein, the investigation died with a subsequent secret grand jury hearing.

Informed that such a hearing had taken place, I wondered who had been investigated. In Massachusetts news that there had even been such a hearing was confined to rumors. Nearly two years later, in 1968, I addressed my questions to the incumbent attorney general of Massachusetts, Elliot Richardson. Had there been an investigation, I asked, and if so, what had come of it? Richardson told me that the investigation had been undertaken by his predecessor, Edward Brooke, and he was not at liberty to give out information on it. But, he assured me, I need not worry, since Joseph Kosow was then "old material." Apparently I was to forget that Rubinstein was still in office and that Kosow's kingdom was still expanding.

Richardson admitted only that there had been an investigation. Neither he nor anyone else would say whether any action had been taken concerning the checks from Kosow to Rubinstein. A reporter for the *Record American* in Boston, Jean Cole, encountered similar frustration in her efforts to find out what had happened. No one seemed to know anything about the hearing.

Determined to find out about the grand jury investigation with—or, as it turned out, without—the help of either Richardson or the Suffolk County (Boston) court, I continued my search for the facts. Under Massachusetts law, the state attorney general can institute a special grand jury investigation. Upon finding evidence of criminal action, the grand jury refers its finding to the county prosecutor for action. Such special investigations are listed on the grand jury docket as "Commonwealth vs. John Doe."

By reading through every page of the grand jury docket, listing cases and witnesses for the three-year period from 1964 to 1967, I found, under the date of December 12, 1966, this entry: "Commonwealth vs. John Doe. Witnesses (1) Joseph Kosow, 200 Bald Pate, (2) Joseph Carver, 122 Clinton." No cause for action was noted. Dr. Rubenstein, the key figure, had not been called; Paul Wallins, who had made the accusation, had not been called. Dr. Samuel Levey, who said he had been offered bribes, was not called, nor were his superiors in the health department. The newspaper that had tried to track down information concerning the hearing was given no notice of the hearing or of its outcome. Only in the grand jury list of witnesses was the slight, vestigial evidence to be found.

What force had shut off the investigation? Only the then attorney general, Edward Brooke, could have answered.

A subcommittee staff member thought the answer might lie with campaign contributions. The subcommittee had been told that the Brooke-for-senator campaign had received a $150,000 loan from the City Bank and Trust Company (whose president, Ruben Epstein, had participated with Dr. Rubenstein in Kosow's Florida deal) and a $20,000 contribution from Joseph Kosow's associate, Dr. David Levy, now owner of the Neponset View Nursing Home. Campaign files confirmed the names of the donors, though the amounts listed were smaller. The files also turned up several other Kosow associates as Brooke contributors. Another factor in Brooke's apparent reluctance to pursue the investigation may have been the presence on his staff of two assistant attorneys general who were linked to the Kosow interests.

The reluctant investigators went on to higher office, Brooke as U.S. Senator and Richardson, most recently, as U.S. Attorney General. The experience of Dr. Samuel Levey, who testified to the attempted bribes, was different.

Dr. Levey took his job seriously from the moment he was appointed; with the idealism of the fresh warrior, he struck at the industry. For a while he was able to close homes unwilling to correct serious violations of the state licensure regulations. As he later described it to me, the nursing homes had been caught sleeping. Eventually, however, the industry mustered its strength and struck back. The battle to enforce standards settled into its normal pattern of violation, citation, promise to correct—followed by another citation and another empty promise. Even inspections returned to their old pattern. Supposedly unannounced, they were in fact known about in advance by the nursing home to be inspected.

After Dr. Levey testified that he not only had been offered bribes but had refused them, the state legislature punished him for his audacity by freezing his pay scale. That had the desired effect: Dr. Levey resigned.

As for Dr. Rubenstein, he retired in 1970, and a party was held in his honor.

Unscathed on the political front, Kosow himself kept expanding his operations. After Massachusetts came Connecticut. A member of the Senate subcommittee staff tried to warn Connecticut in a memo to Senator Abraham Ribicoff:

> There is a great deal more about these people and their operations which should be known by state authorities if they are to be forewarned and forearmed. . . . The Kosow operations in Connecticut are reaching a major scale. . . . I have heard figures as high as 33 for the Connecticut homes in which he is in some way involved. . . . My only concern in this matter, as far as Connecticut goes, is that your officials realize that this is not a routine operation entering the state, but has the potential for becoming a major problem for them.

That was back in 1966. Connecticut did not keep Kosow out, and in 1972 he was reported to be entering New York State. And contrary to Elliot Richardson's statement that he is "old material," Joseph Kosow the moneylender has most recently gotten into the very newest form of the nursing home hustle: the publicly owned chains.

7

Let the Stockholder Beware

THE "FEVERED FIFTY" OF 1969 were not victims of a typhoid epidemic. Not people at all, they were, in Wall Street jargon, a group of nursing home stocks whose arrival on the market had set off a convulsion of greed among promoters, brokers, and investors. Writing of the "fevered fifty" in early 1969, J. Richard Elliott, Jr., of *Barron's* commented that a ". . . kind of frenzy seems to grip the stock market at the merest mention of those magic words 'convalescent care,' 'extended care,' 'continued care.' All euphemisms for the services provided by nursing homes, they stand for the hottest investment around today."

It was quite a change for the nursing home industry. Certainly Mom and Pop never thought their little operation was "the hottest investment around" in their time. The small-time operators, working so hard to steal a dollar here, a hundred there, never aspired to the big-league robbery possible on Wall Street. Nor did the scramble to invest in nursing! homes accord with the poverty-stricken image of itself that the industry continued to present whenever it was lobbying the legislatures for higher rates.

New operators had brought new methods to the industry. The flood of government money that began with Medicaid and Medicare in 1966 had attracted a new breed of profiteer. These men were more likely to be certified public accountants than from the ghetto grocery store that produced Sandy Novak. All they had in common with their predecessors was the desire for profit and the lack of any previous interest in delivering health care. Knowledgeable in the intricacies of tax law and financial manipulation, the newcomers perceived that while the oldtimers had labored to steal thousands, it was now possible to make millions by methods that in most cases were legal.

The newcomers brought two related changes into the industry: the nursing home chain and the "publicly owned" company. Where the shoestring operator bought nursing homes one at a time, men with ready access to capital were able to buy them in wholesale lots. The chain operations grew rapidly; by 1972 an estimated ninety chains owned 12 percent of the nation's nursing homes. As we shall see later in this chapter, many of those chains are interrelated, with the result that ownership and power in this industry is increasingly concentrated in fewer hands.

The next move was "going public"—selling shares in the chains to the public through brokers. The public, which as taxpayer was already paying the industry's high profits on government revenue, was now asked as investor to finance the promoter's desire for still more profits. The bait to the investor was that he, too, could get in on the take—of his own money, that is, since most of it came from the government. The industry arrived on Wall Street loudly proclaiming its own profitability—out of only one side of its mouth, however, for the other side was still telling the state legislatures that the industry needed yet another rate increase to avoid bankruptcy. The stocks were offered to the public at prices far above the customary 17:1 ratio of price to earnings. (New stocks are usually offered at a price no more than seventeen times what the stock is expected to earn in one year per share.) Nonetheless, brokers touted nursing home stocks as sound investments on which, buyers were told, it was possible to earn a return of 20 percent a year. With guaranteed government revenue and the growing number of older people, it did not seem possible for the investor to lose.

Some observers saw a redeeming social purpose in the sale of stock to the public. This new source of capital would pay off the old high-cost debt in Kosow-style loans and would provide the industry with a stable financial base. With new money and new operators, the industry could dispense with its "bad guys"—embarrassing personalities like Eugene Woods. None of that was to happen. What the industry got was Eugene Woods in a pinstripe suit.

The boom was as brief as it was hot. By 1971 most of the "fevered fifty" stocks had fallen far below their high points of a couple of years earlier. Many shirts had been lost, though few belonged to those who had promoted the stocks. As a Chicago nursing home operator observed, "When these chains get into trouble and go broke, the owners are still rich. It is the public that has gone broke." The claim that the industry was highly profitable was, of course, accurate; what no one said, even in the fine print, was that the promoters had no intention of cutting the investors in on the take. For the investor, as ignorant as he was eager for profit, it was like going spearfishing in a school of sharks. It was always possible to surface unscathed with a fish on his spear, but he was in the water with creatures who were faster and stronger than he, and quite willing to gobble him up along with his fish. The public as investor was playing the same role in the industry as it did as taxpayer—that of victim.

The case of the Four Seasons chain offers classic proof that a roller-coaster ride ends at the bottom. Stock in Four Seasons Nursing Centers of America was first offered at $11,00 a share. It shot up to a peak of $181.50, then shot down just as fast, and by the time trading in the stock was suspended, it was selling for $.50 a share. The chain went into bankruptcy proceedings in a federal court that was soon to be labeled "scandal ridden."

As the "disinterested" trustee to administer the firm, a federal court in Oklahoma appointed a paid consultant to Four Seasons; furthermore, a judge who made one of the decisions in the case was the father of a Four Seasons lawyer. The proceedings produced testimony to the political clout of Four Seasons in at least one state. The chain had managed to get from the state of Ohio an unsecured loan of $4 million, later described as illegal by the state auditor. (Ohio did better than most investors: the state got one-third of its money back when a Four Seasons home in Ohio was sold—to a former business associate of Eugene Woods.) Four Seasons stock was used, along with that of another firm involved in the Ohio loan, to make a loan to a New York investment firm (Hayden Stone)—a purpose pretty far removed from nursing homes. Finally, in December 1972 eight people—three officers of Four Seasons, two partners and an employee of its accountants (Arthur Andersen), two former officers of a brokerage firm (Walston)—were indicted on charges that included defrauding the investors and making false statements to the Securities and Exchange Commission. According to the indictments, the officers phonied Four Seasons figures, raising the apparent profits to run up the stock's price, and the accountants certified the figures. When the stock began to fade, the indictment charged, the officers bailed out by selling their own stock through secret accounts at the brokerage house. That left the other investors holding the bag with next to nothing in it. As matters stand as of this writing, the average stockholder may get back something like 10 cents on the dollar. The loss to investors of $200 million was described by the prosecutor as a record for stock-fraud indictments—pretty good for an industry that had not even been on Wall Street a few years earlier. (Four Seasons, though down, is not out: at last report, it was making a come-back under the name of Anta Corporation.)*

The Four Seasons fiasco is discounted as an exception by the industry. Certainly Four Seasons was the most spectacular boom-and-bust in nursing home stocks and the fact that accountants and brokers as well as promoters were actually indicted puts it in a class by itself. However, the public records demonstrate that Four Seasons is not the only chain that has exploited both the public as investor and the public as taxpayer. Those records are mainly documents that companies wanting to sell stock must file with the Securities and Exchange Commission. The documents, though far from adequate to protect the investor, do provide a wealth of information. The result is that we know a lot more about nursing home swindles involving stocks than we do about the secret owners or the moneylenders.

The public is usually told, in the prospectus that accompanies the offering of stock, that the proceeds of the sale of stock will be used to pay off heavy existing debts (typically, lower-position mortgages) on the homes the chain now owns and to build or acquire new homes. Less debt and more homes will make for more profit. Always, the potential investor is reminded that the company's continued good health is dependent on continued government revenue. If government rocks the boat, the company and its investors will be swamped. Somewhere in the documents filed at the SEC one will, more often than not, learn that the owners of the chain also own other companies, visually in finance and construction, that do business with the chain.

The annual reports filed with the SEC in later years

---

* Jack L. Clark, the former president of Four Seasons, who was charged with making $10 million for himself out of the operation, has since pleaded guilty. He was sentenced to one year in prison, making him eligible for parole in four months; not a cent in fines was imposed. Assuming he is released after the minimum time served, the sentence works out to one month in jail for each fraudulently acquired $2.5 million.

show how far practice varies from the promises contained in the prospectus. First, the original owners take a healthy cut of the investors' money for themselves. Their own stock in the original company is revalued, when going public, at a much higher price; the difference is sometimes astronomical. If the promoters buy stock in the new company, they allow themselves to buy it at a much lower price than the investor pays for the same stock—and sometimes they sell some of their own stock to the investors at inflated prices. So far the investor has enriched the promoters, but not the company or himself.

The investors' money is rarely used for the promised purposes. The excessive debt is seldom paid off; the homes continue to carry second and third mortgages at high interest rates—mortgages often held by a finance company that belongs to the promoters. As for the promised new homes, often they are not built, or if they are, the job is typically done, at a very high price, by the promoters' own construction company.

In these two ways profits are siphoned off into the promoters' other companies, where the take does not have to be shared with the public investor. During the shift of ownership to the new public company, the paper value of the nursing homes is increased, which will push up the reimbursement rate paid by government, as well as increase the value of the stock. What is left of the money put up by the investors is typically used for a purpose not mentioned in the prospectus—to buy up other businesses that frequently have nothing to do with nursing homes or health care generally.

Nothing has changed, except on the surface, as a result of the growth of the chains that sell stock to the public. The taxpayer is still being taken by high profits and inflated costs, but now some taxpayers are paying dues a second time as investors. As for the patients, nothing much has changed for them, either. It is true, as the apologists say, that patients in a chain nursing home are likely to be housed in a building that is newer and shinier than the usual home. But the façade does not determine what goes on inside, where the patients are. Absentee ownership is no asset to patient care. Where a Sanford Novak is at least present in the homes he owns, the chain owners are a thousand miles away, dreaming up new financial coups. Nothing could be further from their minds than the patients they never see—though their actions in large measure determine the quality of the patients' lives. Certainly I have seen as much unnecessary suffering in chain-owned homes as in any other kind.

The case of Charles Wick and United Convalescent Hospitals illustrates the basic strategies of the nursing home chain promoter. Charles Wick is easily the most respectable nursing home operator to have appeared so far in the pages of this book. I knew something about Wick's career before I met him, for my husband and he had attended school together from kindergarten through the University of Michigan. A poor boy, he had musical talent, energy, and intelligence, all of which he put to good use. He became a millionaire as a manager of entertainers, and at forty he retired. He emerged again to enter the nursing home business, and was now president of United Convalescent Hospitals.

Interested in this sequence of events, I went to California to interview him. Sitting in his sumptuous home in Beverly Hills, gazing out at the swimming pool, listening to his articulate explanations, I reflected that the business had come a long way from Sandy Novak grubbing for his money in the Cleveland ghetto. Charles Wick was an officer in the American Nursing Home Association; he was consulted by HEW. He had gotten into the business, he told me, because of what he had seen when he had placed someone in a nursing home. He was determined to improve patient care, he said, and in pursuit of that goal he had spent $10 million without earning a cent in profit. It all sounded as beautiful as our Beverly Hills surroundings, and at the moment I was tempted to believe him.

Back at the SEC files, I pieced together a totally different picture of Mr. Wick and United Convalescent Hospitals. The main difference between him and Sandy Novak, I soon realized, was that Novak was more frank about his business methods. As I worked my way through the SEC documents, I learned that United Convalescent Hospitals was a very good thing for Wick, but not for the taxpayer or investor or patient. Here is some of the information available from those files:

When Wick and his associates went public in 1968, United Convalescent owned eight nursing homes and had two more under development. In 1964, when the company was originally formed, Wick and his associates had put up $1,123,800 for one million shares—$1.12 a share. By 1967, after three straight years of losses, the shares had a paper value of $.36. Now, only a few months later, the public was offered the opportunity to buy 529,260 shares—at $10.00 a share. The effect of this infusion of new money would be to make everyone's shares, the public's as well as the original investors', worth $3.39. Not bad for the original owners. Their shares would now be worth triple what they paid for them ($1.12) and thirty times their current value of $.36. The public, on the other hand, would pay (at $10.00) three times what the shares were now supposed to be worth ($3.39) and nine times what the original investors had paid ($1.12).

Of the approximately $5 million raised by the sale of stock, $1.5 million was used to pay off loans the original investors had advanced to the various homes. Some of these loans had been made to provide the 10 percent owner's down payment required in order to get FHA financing. (More than $1 million of the loans came from Mapleton Capital Corporation, which belonged to Charles Wick.) According to FHA rules, such loans could be repaid only out of surplus cash, after all other liabilities were paid off. But those loans, which were to be paid last, were in fact paid first, and most of the money went to Wick's company.

The pattern of raising the value of homes by paper transactions, in order to increase government revenue and improve the company's financial image, is evident in the SEC files on United Convalescent. (Medicare only allows an increase in value when the home changes hands, and the creation of United Convalescent provided that opportunity.) The value of the eight homes in operation was increased by an average of $125,000 each, with no evidence that the homes had been expanded or improved. One of the larger increases in paper value occurred with the Los Angeles Convalescent Center. Its original value, in 1965, was about $1.7 million; when it was taken over by the corporation two years later, it was said to be worth $1,985,000.

The prospectus and the annual reports of United Convalescent are full of contradictions and inconsistent figures, never explained to the investor, never challenged by the SEC. One mystery concerns the Sun Ridge Home in Columbus, Ohio. The 1969 annual report informed stockholders that Sun Ridge had been acquired by the corporation. However, two years later public deed and health department records still listed Sun Ridge in the names of the original owners.

Thus the original promoters of United Convalescent had managed, by going public, first to raise the value of their properties so the government had to pay more for patient care, second, they had gotten the public to buy shares in a money-losing enterprise at from three to thirty times (depending on how you figure it) the apparent value of those shares. Perhaps the investors thought the company was going to turn around and make a lot of money. It did not: the company continued to report losses.

An explanation for the earlier losses, before the firm went public, can be found in the SEC files. The profits had been shifted out of the United Convalescent to a series of other enterprises, all owned in whole or in part by Charles Wick. Here are some examples.

Charles Wick's wholly owned Mapleton Enterprises rendered management services to the nursing homes under development and management contracts. As part of its development services, Enterprises, for $745,000, acquired land that it resold to the nursing homes for $855,000; if homes were built on that land the increased figure would thereafter be the basis for Medicare-Medicaid rates to be paid the homes and charges to private patients. Under its management contract, Enterprises received $325,000 for a two-year-plus period, figured on a management cost of $10 per bed per month.

During that same period, Wick's lending company, Mapleton Capital, received $23,000 in interest payments, while Financial Systems Corporation, in which Wick held an indirect 50 percent interest, received $125,000 for rendering financial services to the homes. And a construction company wholly owned by Charles Wick received $3,070,000 to build homes for the corporation.

One exhibit at the SEC demolishes any illusion that the FHA's involvement controls construction costs. That exhibit is a development contract between one of the homes, Fort Pierce Nursing, and Wick's Mapleton Enterprises. The exhibit states:

> [The development company] shall receive such amounts-allowable by the Federal Housing Administration in fees and direct cost reimbursement. . . . Further as compensation ... in addition to any Federal Housing Administration allowable fees and direct cost reimbursement, [the company] shall receive an amount equal to ten percent of the total cost of the project.

Wick's services to the company appeared in still other areas. A company in which he was an officer helped his

166 · Tender Loving Greed

nursing home process their mortgage applications to the FHA—a service for which the company received a fee of $55,000, to be paid out of nursing home revenue. Another firm in which Wick had an indirect 50 percent interest was paid $5,000 for its services as a real estate broker in connection with the acquisition of a San Francisco site; and as the prospectus declares, if other sites then being considered in Florida and Georgia were acquired, the realty commissions would rise by $44,000.

Within a year, the company moved into other fields. It bought a home health-care company, a therapy company, an optical dispensing company, and finally a pharmaceutical business in Louisiana owned by R. Lewis Rieger, who, the stockholders were told, was "strong . . . seasoned in the pharmaceutical business and growth oriented." However, the reports that United Convalescent filed with the SEC in connection with the purchase of Rieger show that company losing money in two of the last three years when reports were submitted.

After its first two years as a public company, United Convalescent continued to lose money. But this, of course, did not mean no money was being made in connection with that enterprise. When Charles Wick told me he had invested $10 million in nursing homes and gotten nothing back, he did not tell about his other corporations that were making money doing business with United Convalescent. By selling stock to the public, Wick and his associates had gotten back the money they had originally invested. (Those associates, incidentally, included Joseph Cole, currently treasurer of the Democratic National Committee, and entertainers Pat Boone, Gene Kelly, and Frances Langford. Boone owns a nursing home in Boca Raton, Florida, which has a lease arrangement with United Convalescent.) Yet the corporation's losses could be paraded before the public as a justification for higher rates, and Wick himself could testify before a Senate subcommittee in 1970 that "many [homes] are on the verge of going broke. Medicare and Medicaid are not reimbursing them for their true costs, and profits are nonexistent." (Because it was losing money, United Convalescent was subsequently merged with another chain, Hill Haven. Wick received a three-year contract at $60,000 a year as chairman of the board of the expanded Hill Haven chain. Six months later, in June 1972, Wick resigned, without explanation to the stockholders.)

California, home of Charles Wick, provides us another example of the draining off of profits from the company in which the public has invested. This one resulted in the conviction of the chief officers of a nursing home chain bearing the odd name of Convalariums of America.

The president and chairman of the board of Convalariums of America, Fred E. Elg, along with the executive vice-president and treasurer, Harold Kirsch, were found guilty of fraudulent activities in California in 1971. Elg and Kirsch had set up six dummy corporations, which rendered phony invoices, at inflated prices, to Convalariums. These invoices were paid by Convalariums, and payment to the actual suppliers, at lower prices, was made by the dummy corporations, with Elg and Kirsch collecting the difference.

Elg resigned from Convalariums in the fall of 1970. In fulfillment of the SEC requirement that companies must file periodic reports noting major changes, notice of his resignation was duly filed, with no reference to the felony charge against him. Nor were stockholders of Convalariums told why their company had taken on new leadership.* The investors might not have cared if their executives had been caught in the pursuit of profit for the investors. Certainly they would have been interested to know that their leaders had been siphoning off money that might otherwise have gone to the investors in the form of dividends.

---

*Convalariums later changed its name to C-V America, Inc. It is typical of the industry that chains frequently change their names—a tacit acknowledgment, it would seem, that those names have no value in goodwill.

Another publicly owned company, Metrocare Enterprises, is a classic example of how the cost of homes is inflated. Oakview Nursing Home, in Sayreville, New Jersey, was valued at $832,381 in 1968. The following year, Metro-care bought Oakview for $2,250,000. Nothing had been done to Oakview to make it worth more than twice its value of a year earlier.* Its owners, however, did very well for themselves out of the Metrocare promotion. Frank Gabriel, half-owner of Oakview (50 shares at $100 a share), got a remarkable return on his $5,000 investment: he received a cash payment of $801,194 from the proceeds of the sale of stock, and was also given the right to buy 15,000 shares of Metrocare stock at $.15 a share—at the same time that the public was being asked to pay $12.00 a share. For Frank Gabriel, at least, the nursing home business is very healthy.

Metrocare subsequently registered for stock offerings twice more, the second time to finance the building of condominiums in New Jersey, and most recently has embarked upon an especially ambitious project with its formation of Senior Advocates International, Inc. In a promotional brochure for this new organization, Metrocare identifies itself as "developer of planned retirement communities . . . operator of health care facilities . . . and provider of consulting and management services to the medical industry." SAI's avowed purpose is to serve as "an advocate for the fulfillment of the unique needs and interests of all Americans 50 or older," and its "advisory committee" consists primarily of various philanthropic groups of excellent repute. Benefits offered to prospective members include: "A low-cost health insurance policy; specially priced travel programs; a subscription to 'Senior Advocate' magazine; discount automobile rentals; pharmaceutical products by mail at low prices;

*As an example of the sloppiness that is permitted by the Securities and Exchange Commission, Oakview reported different income and profit figures for the same year on two documents filed with the SEC in connection with the sale of Metrocare stock to the public.

independent hotel packages at attractive rates; representation of your legislative interests." SAI has arranged, the brochure continues, "to provide these services through the facilities of some of the most prestigious companies in the country. Insurance through ITT Family Security Sales Corp., a subsidiary of International Telephone and Telegraph . . . pharmaceutical products through Vitamin Quota Inc. . . . independent travel packages arranged through TV Travel, Inc., a subsidiary of Top Value Enterprises, using facilities of Hilton Hotels Corporation . . . rental car discounts from Hertz and National." And the cost for all this? An annual fee of $5, or $13 for three years. (Blocked off enticingly in the brochure is an additional offer of information, upon request, about parent firm Metrocare's health care facilities.)

I had not been studying the stock-selling chains for long before I ran across the trails of two characters whom we met in earlier chapters: Dr. Bernard Bergman, the secret owner, and Joseph Kosow, the moneylender. I was not surprised. One could hardly expect two such expert sharpshooters to overlook so inviting a target as the investing public.

Dr. Bergman was first on the scene. As noted in Chapter 5, Bergman's Medic-Home went public in 1968, and some of the proceeds were used to buy Freezie, the firm whose product was so mysterious that it could not be identified from any of the available records. Here I shall add only one more note on Bergman's corporation and its investors.

Besides buying Freezie, Medic-Home investors were told in the original prospectus that the company intended to use their money to develop a 150-bed nursing home in Columbus, Ohio. The president of the company, Samuel Klurman, in the 1968 annual report to the stockholders, reported happily on the home under construction in Columbus. In his 1969 annual report, the Columbus facility had been placed on the list of the Medic-Home Health Centers as an operating business. A stockholder, perusing his annual report, would have no reason not to count 150 additional beds as among his company's assets. Columbus officials, however, could disillusion him. They report that the company never applied for an operating license until August 1970, almost two years after the company had assured the stockholder that the building was under construction. They say that the building first opened its doors in September 1970—nine months after the annual report listed it as among the homes then in operation.

In the leadership of Medic-Home were three people closely connected with a firm called the First Connecticut Small Business Investment Company. Its officers were part of Medic-Home management, and the bank was a principal stockholder in the company. First Connecticut provides our first evidence of a connection of Kosow with Bergman. The connection is indirect, because the names of Kosow and Bergman seldom appear in the records of their enterprises. The connection is through mortgages. Kosow-dominated management companies and nursing homes with a Kosow connection have assigned their mortgages to the Bergman-linked First Connecticut.

Kosow is involved in other chains. He appears through some of his associates in connection with a chain called Geri-Care (which has recently changed its name to Lifestyle Companies). The prospectus states that money raised by the sale of stock in Geri-Care will be used in part to pay off a loan to one Hyman Temkin, who was part owner of one of Kosow's investment companies. Among the exhibits in the SEC files are two agreements between another Kosow associate and the president of Geri-Care, Dr. Sydney Nathans (Kosow's name does not appear in the prospectus). At that time, 1969, the SEC knew of Temkin's connection with Kosow, and had already investigated Kosow himself (for the stock manipulations that resulted in his conviction, later reversed). Yet the SEC did not insist that the prospectus warn the potential investor of the company's connections to Kosow.

The Geri-Care prospectus attracted the attention of the Senate Finance Committee when it was investigating nursing homes in 1969. The committee observed that Geri-Care was buying homes for much more than they had cost to build, and it was concerned about the effect that the establishment of a new and higher base for depreciation might have on Medicare rates. The committee recognized a dangerous trend in the growth of chains, but it did not really grasp the significance of the "Kosow-touch" mortgages on some Geri-Care homes which exceeded the original worth of those homes. Then-Senator John Williams of Delaware noted an evident conflict of interest: a director of Geri-Care, John J. Budds, was also director of Medicare operations for the Travelers Insurance Company, which audits nursing home bills for Medicare. (Budds's name was later dropped by Geri-Care.)

Senator Williams also pointed out how extraordinarily well the president of Geri-Care, Dr. Sydney Nathans, was doing out of the sale of stock. Dr. Nathans originally held all the stock in Geri-Care, with the value of his investment figured at $305,000. In going public, he sold some of his stock and thus recouped his investment and made a profit of $485,000, while the stock that he retained jumped in value to $1,322,000. In addition, part of the proceeds was used to pay off his loans to the company of $100,000.

During its first six months as a public company, Geri-Care tightened its bonds to Kosow by acquiring two homes built and managed by him, and carrying his mortgages. The corporation had also bought homes in Connecticut from Kosow's nominee, Charles Brennick, in a deal that included an agreement that Brennick would add 1,092 beds to the homes at a cost of $12,000 per bed—a high price compared to Medic-Home's costs of $5,000 per bed at that same time.

(A startling departure from the health-care business was revealed in the corporation's report to its stockholders in 1970 that it had advanced $395,000 to the D. B. Wesson Company, Inc., of Monson, Massachusetts, to complete the tooling for a "unique handgun" with interchangeable barrels. It had also acquired an option to purchase the Wesson Company. Stockholders were assured that the handgun had already received an overwhelmingly favorable response from both sporting and law-enforcement interests.)

Another large chain in which Joseph Kosow is involved is Century Convalescent Centers, which went public in November 1969. (Century recently changed its name to National Health Services.) According to its original prospectus, the chain's executive offices were in Beverly Hills, California. Its thirty-seven homes, representing 3,989 beds, were located in California, Florida, Massachusetts, Georgia, and Alabama, with each of the four homes in Massachusetts connected directly or indirectly with Kosow. The principal stockholders were listed as Dr. and Mrs. David A. Levy, current owner of the Neponset View Nursing Home, which figured in the last chapter. As Century grew, its holdings spread through many regions, and its history shows the interlocking connections among nursing home operations, including some of its directors' links with other chains.

Century established ties, through a mortgage, to Dr. Bernard Bergman's Medic-Home Enterprises, by purchasing the operating company of the Martin Nursing Home through a stock transfer deal. (That home had been built by Joseph Kosow, and managed and financed by him; in the stock transfer, some shares were to be donated to his brother, Jack Kosow.) The Martin Home had been encumbered by several mortgages, a fourth mortgage being held by the First Connecticut Small Business Investment Company, a principal in Medic-Home Enterprises.

In March 1970 Century acquired two homes in the

Chicago area, the Austin and the Evergreen, in return for 120,000 shares of Century stock valued at $10 per share. Of those shares, 87,000 went to one of the owners, Shelton Shefferman. (He had been in a labor consultant business. When in 1957, Dave Beck, the Teamster leader, was indicted for criminal activities in the labor field, one of the counts against him involved his accepting the assistance of Shelton Shefferman in evading his income taxes over a period of some ten years.) In July 1970 Shefferman became a director and vice-president of Century and the company's midwestern regional manager. Six months later Century sold the 162-bed Evergreen home for which Shelton Shefferman had received 39,429 shares of Century stock to the Golden Age Nursing Centers, of Chicago, for $175,000. This was a remarkably low price, since the home had been valued at $552,000 ten months before. The president of the Golden Age Centers and the holder of 50 percent of the stock in that bargain purchase was—Shelton Shefferman.

In 1971 the Century chain picked up the leases on several nursing homes in Maryland, one located in Montgomery County. The county health department had difficulty trying to identify the ownership and officers or even the address of the corporation's headquarters. When county personnel asked Century's eastern representative about Norman Geller, whom they thought to be the responsible person, they were assured that Geller had severed connections with the company. The address for the eastern division was, the representative reported, 1505 Commonwealth Avenue, Boston. It was most unlikely that the Maryland health officials would recognize the Commonwealth Avenue address as being that of both Norman Geller and Joseph Kosow. Nor would it be common knowledge in Maryland that on the third floor of 1505 Commonwealth are three offices: MetPath, a laboratory company that does work for health-care institutions; the office of Geller and Kosow; and another office—that of Century Convalescent Homes. These three groups occupy the entire third floor, sharing common conference rooms.

Individuals involved in the nursing home business with Kosow turned up again in another huge nursing home chain, Health Care Corporation. It registered in 1968 to go public, then withdrew its registration; it reregistered in 1970 and withdrew again. When it originally registered, it claimed assets of $16 million and a total of 15 homes in operation. Two years later it claimed to have 188 subsidiaries, of which 114 were nursing homes, and 74 dental and medical supply houses. Its assets totaled $122 million.

So Kosow, the moneylender, is involved in at least three nursing home chains. Those chains in turn are connected with other chains through interlocking directorships, mortgages, and other deals. What this seems to indicate is that, although there are many chains, power in the industry is far more concentrated than it would appear on the surface.

The presence of Bergman and Kosow, the activities of Wick and the others I have described, are clear evidence of what is happening in a significant part of the nursing home industry now that it is selling stock to the public. The usual patterns of beating the government and the taxpayer have been carried over from earlier days: the inflating of apparent costs to raise reimbursement rates, the shifting of profits to other companies. And as usual, the patients must suffer from scrimping and neglect so that profits can be maximized. All that has changed is that the investor has been added to the list of the industry's victims—and that the sums involved have multiplied.

The Securities and Exchange Commission supposedly protects the investor, but in reality it does not accomplish that purpose. The documents that companies selling shares to the public must file with the SEC are a goldmine of information. Most of the evidence detailed in this chapter comes from those files. However, I was able to dig it out because I was willing to spend weeks in Washington going through the documents—and because I was familiar enough by then with the industry to know what to look for. Few investors would be willing to make that effort, and few would be knowledgeable enough to detect the hustles hidden in innocent-seeming statistics. The information in any case is not sufficient to determine what is really going on. Nothing in the prospectus of a company that has gone public gives a breakdown for each nursing home, the cost of care, the original cost per bed, the number of mortgages, and hence the new cost per bed. Only a consolidated financial statement accompanies the registration statement. The exhibits frequently assure the reader of accompanying statements, but too often those attachments are missing. Examples of missing documents that disturbed me because of the potential for abuse were statements about leases. Several agreements registered within the exhibits will state, "Attached is a copy of the lease." The lease is not there, though it may be the crucial information that makes the exhibit intelligible.

No investor reading that there are X number of dollars of assets tied up in second and third mortgage liabilities can know whether a principal in the company indirectly holds those profitable mortgages. Not only is the investor in the dark, but so is the Securities and Exchange Commission. And since the breakdown of expenses is seldom given, neither the investor nor the SEC knows if the rent was taking an abnormally large share of expenses for a particular home. Even in those rare files when the figures are given in a sketchy accounting, discrepancies can be found within the prospectus.

Nursing homes are new on the market; the civil servant has not readjusted his eyeshade to the light of a new set of problems. Securities and Exchange has not discovered what information should be required to substantiate claims made in a nursing home prospectus. An industry regulated by state and federal requirements and supported primarily by federal and state taxes, vested with a public interest, is treated virtually the same as any other business.

One useful and easy change that the SEC could make has to do with the reporting of nursing home inspections. If the company's homes are in violation of state or federal regulations, they may lose their licenses—which would obviously affect the investor. But the SEC does not require the prospectus to contain any information on the results of inspections. If the last inspection report were required to be attached to the prospectus, many an investor might well refuse to buy.

Finally, before leaving the subject of nursing home chains, let us visit a place that neatly sums up the message of this chapter. The Encino Hospital in Encino, California, is owned by Beverly Enterprises, a big nursing home chain that has been spreading into other parts of the health-care business. The president of Beverly, Roy Christensen, is a CPA who, according to Barren's, has made $10 million on an investment of $5,700 in the chain. Beverly encourages the doctors who serve its patients to invest in its operations, perhaps on the assumption that the doctors will discern the connection between a full nursing home or hospital and the health of their investments. The assumption appears sound. So interested are the physicians at the Encino Hospital, according to a report by Roger Rapoport in the December 1972 *Harper's,* that in a lounge next to the surgical suite they keep a television tuned to a UHF business channel that reports, among other stock market news, the current status of their investment in the Beverly empire.

With all that we have seen since nursing homes began selling their stock, we must conclude that the process of going public has only served to broaden the opportunity to practice the old nursing home swindle under a new cloak of legitimacy.

8

"Highly Profitable Ancillary Services"

A WALL STREET ANALYST, writing about the American Medical Enterprises chain, observed that: "An important part of the company's expansion program is centered around adding highly profitable ancillary services at several facilities."

Ancillary services, and they are indeed highly profitable, include in the nursing home industry everything that is not part of the regular budget of the home. The most important among such services are drugs, physicians and other health professionals, laboratory tests, and ambulance services. The services are ordered by the nursing home, and the government payment goes directly to the supplier.

The sale of drugs for nursing homes is the biggest, and for the alert swindler, the most lucrative of ancillary services. Medicaid alone pays out an estimated $200 million a year for drugs for its nursing home patients. From the evidence already accumulated about this business, it is a fair estimate that at least half of that bill is padding: that is, if only the needed drugs were ordered, and if the price was right, the government would be paying out less than half what it pays now—and patients who are now overdrugged would be healthier.

Evidence of corruption, collusion, and theft in the nursing home-drug business has been laid out in detail in a series of exposes in several parts of the country. The General Accounting Office reported on drug-nursing home abuses in California and Ohio; California's Department of Justice did its own investigation; New York City periodically learns of scandals in drugs and other ancillary services. My own study of Medicaid records in Ohio found the same conditions, as did another private study in Minnesota. All these investigations agreed that the government is being charged too much for too many drugs, that many of the drugs for which it pays are unnecessary, and that many are, in fact, never delivered. Here are the main ways in which the government is swindled in the drug business.

It begins with the kickback. It is common practice for nursing homes to require pharmacies supplying them with drugs to give them a kickback. (Kickbacks are also found in other ancillary services.) According to the chief inspector of the California State Board of Pharmacy, Joseph J. Santoro, the average kickback is 25 percent of what the pharmacy charges the nursing home (or, in reality, the government). Sometimes the kickback is paid in cash, other times in more unusual ways: buying a car for the nursing home operator or paying his way on his vacation. One pharmacy paid two nursing homes $4,400 a year supposedly to maintain "drug supply rooms": the rooms turned out to be broom closets. The presence of those closets permitted the homes to obtain a higher rate from Medicare on the grounds that they were offering an extra service. To speed their profitable transactions, one nursing home has a direct phone line to its favored pharmacy.

The kickback is logical from the point of view of the pharmacist. The nursing home is an excellent customer. If, as is usually the case, the home gives all its trade to one pharmacist, it is guaranteeing him a large amount of business at the top price (often more than the top price). Anyone bringing in that kind of business would be entitled to demand a discount. But the nursing homes do not ask for a discount, which would have to be passed on to those who ultimately pay the bill—the taxpayers. Instead, the operator extracts a kickback, the government is charged the full price, and the operator and the pharmacist pocket the difference. That difference, judging from the California figure, is around $50 million a year. Not surprisingly, then, there is a trend to common ownership of nursing homes and pharmacies (and other ancillary businesses), particularly on the part of the fast-buck nursing home chain promoters: if you own them both, it keeps the business advantages all in the family.

Instead of getting a discount, the government frequently pays a price higher than the going rate. Although the nursing home is buying drugs in bulk, Medicaid is often charged more than the person who buys at retail. That is, if you walk in off the street and buy a single prescription, you are likely to pay less than Medicaid has to pay for bulk purchases. According to the California investigation, that is the practice of the "vast majority" of pharmacies in the Los Angeles area—and the GAO found the same thing in Ohio. In that state, pharmacies are paid cost plus 50 percent for prescriptions to nursing homes. That would seem to be a healthy profit margin, but evidently it was not good enough for many suppliers, for the GAO found the pharmacies it studied to be charging Medicaid markups that averaged 159 percent for Lanoxin, and 248 for digoxin; the record was set by a pharmacist who marked up his Lanoxin by 1,650 percent.

The difference, or lack of difference, between brand name and generic drugs provides another profitable opportunity for the nursing home in collusion with the pharmacist. Many widely used drugs appear in two forms: under a brand name and under a generic, or chemical, name. As everyone should know by now, the drugs are identical in all but name and—spectacularly—in price. One example: The brand-name drug Seconal cost $18.30 per thousand at a time when it was also available, under the generic name secobarbital, for $4.00 a thousand. Nembutal is a drug commonly used by nursing homes. At the same time that the average prescription cost $1.95 for twenty-nine capsules ($.067 a capsule), it was available as pentobarbital for $2.25 a thousand capsules ($.002 a capsule, about one-thirtieth the brand-name price). Here again is an excellent opportunity for the nursing home and the pharmacy. The least imaginative of hustlers will insist that the home buy brand-name drugs, keeping up the price to the pharmacy and the kickback to the nursing home. With a bit more imagination they will bill the government for the brand-name drug and in fact supply the cheaper generic equivalent, pocketing the difference. If they are still bolder, as we shall see later in this chapter, they will bill for the brand-name drug—and not give the patient anything at all, thus raising their profit to the ideal of 100 percent.

The cost to the taxpayer of paying for brand-name drugs is considerable. The New York City Bureau of the Budget calculated in 1972 that Medicaid in that city alone would save $1.8 million a year by using generic drugs. The GAO has pointed out to HEW (with no result) that the government could save $41.4 million a year through the use of generic drugs.

A related practice is that of using prescription drugs paid for by the government instead of drugs that the nursing home is supposed to supply without cost. I have noticed, for example, that nursing homes commonly use as a pain-killer the prescription drug Darvon, instead of aspirin. Aspirin is part of the home's normal supplies. Its cost is included in the home's per diem rate, like food or linens, and cannot be billed separately. When a home substitutes Darvon for aspirin, therefore, the effect is to save the home's having to buy aspirin—at great cost, of course, since Darvon is far more expensive than aspirin, although according to the Federal Drug Administration, it is no more expensive to manufacture than aspirin.

At its Minneapolis hearing in late 1971, the U.S. Senate Subcommittee on Long-Term Care heard expert testimony on drug abuse discovered during an investigation of approximately one-fourth of all Minnesota nursing homes. Daphne H. Krause, director of the Minneapolis Age and Opportunity Center, called attention to the lack of adequate controls over drugs in nursing homes. An affidavit from a nursing home employees charged that when patients died, their unused drugs were collected in large cardboard cereal boxes. Another witness said, "Sometimes they wouldn't even take a patient's name off a medicine bottle; they'd just paste another patient's name over it and give them to the other patients. . . . They're getting rich doing this kind of thing." Others told of escalating costs for drugs when private patients, their own resources exhausted, had to be moved to Medicaid. Thereupon, vitamins for which private patients paid $8.00 suddenly cost $18.00; Vaseline, which the private patient purchased for $.49, then cost Medicaid $1.50.

So far we have been describing frauds against the taxpayer that do not necessarily affect the patients, except to the extent that the padding of nursing home costs affects those patients who pay their own way. There is, however, another aspect of the drug business that has a tragic effect on nursing home patients, and that is overdrugging.

Anyone who has spent time in nursing homes is all too familiar with the overdrugged patient: sitting passively, vacant of expression, seeming to sleep with his eyes open. Patients are drugged for the convenience of the management. A person who is tranquilized is less likely to struggle against the cruelty or indifference of the staff; they can do with him as they please. One nursing home operator in California said it was her practice to give a tranquilizer to each new patient as soon as he entered the home. This, she said, was to "make him feel at home"; to feel at home in that home, it seems, means to keep quiet.

Ralph Nader's nursing home raiders published in 1971 their evidence that overdrugging of patients is widespread, that some prescriptions are renewed for years without review by a physician, and that, in some homes, patients have been used as guinea pigs for the testing of new drugs. They cited a retired nursing home administrator's description of over-drugging:

> A layman doesn't know what to look for in a nursing home. He walks in and sees a patient is nice and quiet and he thinks this guy is happy. And the nurse tells him: "This is John. John is one of our best patients. He sits here and watches television."
>
> But you just take a look at John's pupils, and you'll see what condition John is in. John is so full of thorazine that it's coming out his ears. Thorazine—that's a tranquilizer they use. It's a brown pill. It looks like an M & M candy.
>
> The nursing home where I worked kept at least 90 percent of the patients on thorazine all the time. They do it for the money. If they can keep John a vegetable, then they don't have to bother with him. They never have to spend anything to rehabilitate him.

Val Halamandaris, the nursing home expert on the staff of the Senate Special Committee on Aging, has estimated that "fifty percent of the nursing homes in the United States have a serious problem . . . with the amount and number of tranquilizers which are given to patients." Speaking to a 1972 meeting of nursing home administrators, Halamandaris said that a GAO study had turned up the fact that 40 percent of all the drugs paid for by Medicaid are either tranquilizers or sedatives. (Halamandaris's remarks at the meeting were reported in the *Journal of the American College of Nursing Home Administrators*. The journal is "sponsored" by Sandoz Pharmaceuticals, with this acknowledgment: "To Sandoz Pharmaceuticals, makers of Mellaril [Thioridazine] and Hydergine, the college gratefully acknowledges the support which assisted in making this journal a reality." Ironically enough, Mellaril is precisely the kind of drug Halamandaris said was being abused in nursing homes. Sandoz puts out a brochure touting Mellaril for the care of the "agitated geriatric." The cover of the brochure shows three disturbed-looking older people, and the contents advise that the drug can help with "adjustment problems," "behavior problems," "management problems," and "family problems.")

While drugging patients to keep them docile is evidently common in nursing homes, it would be a mistake to assume that all the drugs charged to the government are in fact administered to the patients for whom they were ordered. Given the larcenous relationships between nursing homes and pharmacies, what appears to be overdrugging is likely often to be overbilling. The government, that is, is being billed for drugs that are not delivered, or if delivered, not administered. (Considering the size of the drug orders for individual patients that appear in the records, it is fortunate for many patients that the drugs are not in fact administered to them.) I have been told that the excess drugs for which the government has paid are often resold at a discount to another pharmacy, or sometimes even sold on the street.

I have confirmed the existence of this practice at least in Ohio nursing homes by checking patients' records against Medicaid records. In case after case I have found that the nurse's notes do not report administering to a patient a drug for which Medicaid is paying. When I have compared the purchase records to the nursing home's quarterly evaluations of patients (which record patients' drug needs), I have found that Medicaid is usually paying for more medication—sometimes twice as much—as the patient is recorded as needing.

These discoveries, however, can only be made long after

the fact. Because pharmacies habitually send in their bills months after the supposed delivery of the drugs, and because Medicaid is frequently tardy about paying its bills, it would be impossible for a caseworker or auditor to check current bills against the state of the patient at that time. The fact that it is not done later, which would be better than nothing, is a symptom of lack of interest on the part of the regulators. Medicare records are even more difficult to work with than Medicaid's. Reading the computer printouts that list drug bills and dates makes it obvious, in any event, that the dates are contrived and do not reflect what is actually happening.

The printouts typically list patients as receiving drugs from the day of their arrival in the nursing home—though it must be a rare patient who is both seen by a physician on the day of his arrival and who also receives a prescription drug on that same day. Far more remarkable is the fact that drug deliveries for patients almost always stop exactly one day before death—indicating, if true, remarkably accurate forecasts by the nursing home staff. Obviously, the dates are falsified; the motive doubtless varies according to the nature of the hustles being practiced by a given home and pharmacist. It is common also for a pharmacy to claim to have made three separate deliveries in a single week for a patient, week after week.

One pharmacy and nursing home in Cleveland illustrate the questionable nature of this relationship and a remarkable case of either overdrugging or overcharging. This pharmacy is a one-man operation in which business is conducted in a remote location, open (to nursing homes only) just three days per week. The pharmacist, Gerald Herman, had gotten into trouble with the law twice when he was running a pharmacy that traded with the public. Once he was fined for selling amphetamines without prescription; the second time he was fined and put on probation in connection with a narcotics sale. In his nursing-home-only business, however,

Mr. Herman has made an impressive comeback. He is the leading supplier of drugs for four Cleveland nursing homes, and over a period of seven months in 1970-71 he was collecting from Medicaid an average of $19 per month for each of some 150 Medicaid patients. He also netted an unknown amount from about 160 Medicare and private patients in those homes.

In 1971 the relationship between Mr. Herman's Doral Pharmacy and the Broadview Nursing Home was criticized by a medical review team assigned to survey Medicaid patients in the nursing home. The team report stated that the home's physician, Dr. Robert Backman, failed to note the reasons for drugs administered to patients. The pharmacy was said to produce illegible labels on which the medications are not identified, and dosages and dates are not given.

The record of one Broadview patient's drug account for the year 1970 should, one would think, arouse the professional curiosity of both an auditor and a physician. In the payments to Doral by Medicaid that year, this one patient's case number appeared frequently in the computer printout. To find out why, I requested a copy of the invoices submitted by the Doral Pharmacy over a period of six months.

No one could examine those invoices without the suspicion—indeed, the hope—that the patient for whom they were ordered did not actually receive all the drugs for which Medicaid so generously paid. In the list of two months' charges (October and November 1970) for that eighty-two-year-old lady, one finds these drugs ordered for her (the explanations for the drugs' uses were provided by my own pharmacist): 180 Dulcolax tablets and 10 Dulcolax suppositories (for constipation); 90 Antivert tablets (for dizziness); 150 Elavil tablets (to relieve the symptoms of depression).

This patient's seemingly extraordinary need for drugs changed abruptly at the end of November 1970. From then until April 1971 (the last date for which I have the state record on this patient), she was cut off completely from the

Dulcolax tablets. Over the four-month period from October 1969 to February 1970, 290 Darvon capsules (for the relief of pain) had been purchased for her; then for one year not a single Darvon capsule was ordered, certainly on the face of it an astonishing recovery from pain. Her drug orders were changed, with only the prescriptions for Elavil remaining constant—except for the price. Varying amounts were charged for the same number of tablets of the same strength.

Another Broadview patient suffered a similarly puzzling fate. As a private patient, she was charged by the nursing home for her drugs, the bills being paid by her son. Disturbed by the high costs, the son took her prescriptions elsewhere to be filled. For these, clear orders were written by her own physician and accurate invoices came from the pharmacy. But when the woman eventually went on Medicaid, all logic vanished from her drug bills. The number of different prescriptions multiplied, the frequency of orders and the money spent in her behalf rose sharply, all under the name of a physician unknown to her family.

Physicians and their professional colleagues also have profitable relationships with nursing homes. In many ways the physician holds the key to the nursing home owner's profits. For one thing, his cooperation is needed to cover many of the operator's swindles in ancillary services. The physician also decides who goes to a nursing home and what level of care the patient needs, and therefore what reimbursement rate the home will receive; he signs the prescriptions for all those unneeded drugs. The doctor's signature on a death certificate is required, at least in Ohio, if the operator is to send the body of a deceased patient to his favorite undertaker, instead of having to send the body to the morgue, where evidence of mistreatment may show up. Supposedly the doctor must have seen the patient within three days preceding death, though there is seldom any evidence that he has actually done so. Medicaid rules also require that each patient be under the supervision of a physician who should see him every 30 days.

The physician-nursing home relationship is a two-way street, for the physician himself is an ancillary service for which government is billed ($100 million a year, at a rough estimate, to Medicaid alone for nursing home patients). A physician may be on a retainer at the nursing home, and also able to bill Medicaid and Medicare directly for patient visits. Doctors frequently practice the "gang visit": the physician who, as we mentioned earlier, dashes through the nursing home in a couple of hours, then bills Medicaid for sixty or seventy-five or ninety patient visits. The California investigation found that "overservicing"—billing for nursing home patients for care they did not need and, in many cases, did not get—was enriching doctors at the expense of Medicaid.*

The California doctors also participated in the "healthy patient" racket: helping nursing homes keep their beds filled with easy patients by sending them people who did not need to be in a nursing home at all. In Los Angeles County in one year, county investigators uncovered 1,300 patients who did not need nursing home care.

Not surprisingly, physician abuses are notorious where the doctor owns a nursing home or hospital. As noted earlier, the Four Seasons chain made a practice of inducing local doctors to invest in its new nursing homes; one Colorado doctor said Four Seasons offered to give him stock in a new home if he would guarantee to supply the home with patients. The California report cited this case:

* The investigators found that, for all their Medicaid patients, whether in or outside of nursing homes, thirty-five doctors collected *in just one year* more than $3 million; one physician got $131,000. (His record has probably been topped, however, by the New York doctor who billed Medicaid for $106,000 in the first six months of 1972—and he was only working part-time. One trembles to think what he might have cost the taxpayer had he gone at it full-time.)

One example of unnecessary services in a physician-owned hospital concerns a patient who was hospitalized for 16 days. Ten blood tests, many of them identical, were taken each day the patient was hospitalized. Of the 160 tests taken, not one revealed an abnormal finding. Multiple x-rays of the chest, skull and cervical spine were also taken although here again no abnormality was ever revealed. This type of overservicing was similarly provided to many other patients in this same hospital.*

All that seemed lacking, remembering the Encino Hospital described in the last chapter, was a TV set on which the physician-owner could watch his profits mount with all those unnecessary tests he had ordered.

Dentists, according to the California investigators, are equally aware of their opportunities. "Examination by dentists of patients in nursing homes is a special area where overservicing exists," the report said. In one year eleven dentists collected almost $1 million from Medicaid, a record approaching that of the greediest doctors. It was also California that produced the optometrist, mentioned in an earlier chapter, who tried to bill Medicaid for prescription sunglasses for a blind nursing home patient.

The ambulance is another ancillary service that provides an opening to the alert swindler.

On September 26, 1971, the *New York Times* published a report on fraudulent claims for transportation of patients covered by Medicaid. The city commissioner of investigation, Robert K. Ruskin, complained that the city of New York "may have been defrauded out of millions of dollars" by some of the companies who transport the sick and disabled poor. There was evidence of charges to the city for round trips on behalf of deceased persons, round trips for some who were dead on arrival at a hospital, double billings by

---

* A variant on this racket is the ordering of laboratory tests by the nursing home without the physician's approval and with the probability that he never sees the results.

two companies for the same trip for the same patient, and the like.

The *Times* story had a familiar ring. It recalled Max Strauss's custom of conveying patients in his own automobile at taxicab rates, with added charges for his own time as driver.

Medicaid coverage for ambulance services from a nursing home to a hospital requires that "the patient [be] taken to the nearest hospital equipped to take care of him." But the Alert Ambulance Company of Cleveland—one of some 60 such firms in the Cleveland area—has been regularly paid for conveying patients unnecessarily long distances. This company, favored by many nursing home operators, would regularly send an ambulance across the city from its "headquarters" in an old house on the west side of Cleveland, pick up a patient at the Forest Hills Nursing Home on the east side—a distance of some twenty-five miles one way—then carry the patient across town to the Metropolitan General Hospital on the west side. The trip of fifty miles is about ten times the distance if the nearest ambulance company had been called and the patient taken to the nearest hospital. The Alert Ambulance Company was also found to have billed twice for some pickups or deliveries, but the company's secretary casually explained that double billings are quite common—mistakes, of course. Nor is any explanation forthcoming for ambulance trips ordered for ambulatory persons or for trips with no recorded destination.

State records of payments to Alert for the years 1968-1970 show that this one company was reimbursed for 2,587 trips. This represented about 5 percent of the Medicaid ambulance business for the entire state of Ohio. Billings for individual trips were as high as $167, with the total payments received being $68,222. And these state records, it should be kept in mind, cover only Medicaid: Alert received an additional 80 percent for some 1,700 of these trips by reason of Medicare coverage. There is no public disclosure of Medicare payments to ambulance companies, so that excellent opportunities exist, here and elsewhere, for collecting double reimbursement for services.

One final ancillary service meriting mention is the repeated use by nursing homes of outpatient and emergency facilities at hospitals.

To qualify for Medicare and Medicaid, a home must provide skilled nursing service and have a physician on call at all times. Built into the very definition of an extended-care facility, the category of nursing home required to offer the most medical services, is the requirement that it offer many of the general services provided by a hospital. Patients attended so carefully should not, it seems, need many trips to outpatient clinics, but all too frequently they are sent there even from homes licensed as extended-care facilities. For these often routine examinations, Medicaid pays a fee for the clinic visit, the costs of all tests, and, of course, for the ambulance trip.

The elderly Medicaid patient at Broadview Nursing Home, an extended-care facility, whose startling drug record was cited earlier in this chapter, was, according to official records, visited by a doctor twenty times in four months. But those twenty visits seemed not to have met the patient's need for medical attention. On the third day after the doctor's last visit, she was taken to the outpatient clinic of a hospital for routine tests. In addition, over the years, this same woman has regularly been transported to an outpatient clinic for treatment as a diabetic, with a cost per visit of as much as $75 for the hospital and $56 for the ambulance. The results of the clinic's diagnoses and treatments were not even reported on her medical chart at the nursing home. Later, when her illness seemed to be diagnosed primarily as heart disease, she was taken to the clinic for an electrocardiogram—an inexpensive, frequently used service such as one might properly expect to find in any approved extended-care facility.

The unwarranted use of hospitals by the nursing homes suggests several possibilities. Either nursing homes do not have the facilities they should have, or physicians are not available when needed, or else they are sharing the wealth with friendly hospitals—sending over patients in order to run up the reimbursements. Each hospital visit is, of course, extremely costly to the taxpayers.

The swindles in ancillary services that we have been describing are the most thoroughly documented of all the types of fraud in the nursing home industry. Much more is known about the pharmacist and the physician, for example, than about the secret owners and the moneylenders. It is much easier to prove a case against the providers of ancillary services—because the billing records exist—than it is to prove that a nursing home operator is stealing funds intended for the patients. The reports cited in this chapter document what is happening; any investigating agency can go out tomorrow, if it were so motivated, and easily uncover more evidence proving the same point. If anyone in authority does not know about these swindles, it is because he does not want to know, and if he does not act, it is because he chooses not to act.

Yet government remains inactive. The federal government created, and now tolerates, the administrative separation of its two major programs that makes it easy for a provider to bill both Medicare and Medicaid for the same service. So uninterested is HEW, in fact, that officials do not even know how much Medicaid money is being spent on ancillary services for nursing home patients. It seemed, as of early 1973, to be somewhere around $600 million a year, but HEW officials said that was the roughest kind of estimate.

Government avoids making the most obvious of reforms. HEW's lack of response on the subject of generic drugs is a case in point. As long ago as 1970, the General Accounting Office recommended that HEW act to make pharmacists and physicians substitute generic drugs for their much more expensive brand-name equivalents. The GAO reported that it had discussed the issue with the Food and Drug Administration, which said that it was studying drug efficacy, that the study was a "continuing one" and that "therefore no priority had been established for its completion." Make of that what you can. The office of then Secretary of HEW Elliot Richardson replied to the GAO that it was "in full agreement" on the matter of generic drugs. "However," the response inevitably continued, "we feel that the inseparability of quality from price requires that we make certain that all manufacturers' versions of every drug product available to American patients are in fact safe and effective." Here Secretary Richardson's office was applying to drugs the most basic myth in the nursing home industry: the notion that price and quality are inseparable. The fact that the same chemical is marketed under two names, one costing thirty times as much as the other, tells us nothing at all about the quality; all it tells us is how gullible we are. Similarly, the fact that nursing home rates are going up rapidly does not tell us that the quality of care is improving—it only tells us that the nursing home industry is lobbying (and swindling) successfully. Of course, lobbyists for the drug industry say that price and quality are inseparable; but there is no reason for the rest of us, including the Secretary of HEW, to share that delusion. The HEW response concluded by postponing the danger of action to the fuzzy bureaucratic future: "The problem is considerably more difficult than we had anticipated and will require substantial time and effort to resolve." If HEW chooses to find the problem too "difficult" to act on, it is because the brand-name drug and nursing home industries are vigilant in defending their interests, while the taxpaying public remains silent.

Even where, as in New York City, Medicaid bills are subject to an audit that uncovers many swindles, the offenders are treated with a kindness that the rest of us might envy should we ever get caught breaking the law. New York's Medicaid auditors concentrate on recovering part of the amounts that have been swindled. No providers of ancillary services have gone to jail or even been put out of business. When, in early 1973, the city health department suspended four doctors and six laboratories from doing business with Medicaid for six months, it was a harsh action by comparison to what goes on elsewhere. At that, the health department did not give out the names of the suspended doctors and laboratories.

California managed the unlikely feat of decreasing the efficacy of its regulation. Before Medicaid, each county in California had teams of inspectors who were able to plug at least some of the leaks to .providers of ancillary services. When Medi-Cal, the state's version of Medicaid, came into effect, pumping hundreds of millions of dollars into the business, California turned over auditing of the program to Blue Cross and Blue Shield—and disbanded its local inspection teams. Blue Cross and Blue Shield, themselves part of the health industry, did little to regulate the suppliers whose bills they were paying, and the county authorities had lost what little capacity to act they had once possessed. Similarly, the professional consultants whose prior consent is required before some kinds of services (major dentistry, for example) can be billed to the government, were no longer informed, as they had been before, how much had been charged for the services they had approved. This, the consultants said, "greatly diminished their ability to discover abuses"—obviously so, since it was now possible for the provider to bill for much more work than the consultant had approved. When the California Department of Justice conducted its investigation, it found regulation so lax that it could not even estimate the amount of fraud that was going on. After giving some estimates of fraud under the old system, the investigators delivered themselves of this massive understatement on the effect of less regulation: "It is

therefore highly unlikely that the practice of excessive billing ended with the enactment of the Medi-Cal program."

The statement sums up where we are today. It is "highly
unlikely" that the swindles in ancillary services to nursing
homes will do anything but increase as long as the regulatory
authorities persist in closing their eyes to what is going on.

9

Money Without Profit

THE OPTIMISTIC REFORMER, after viewing the profiteering that goes on in the nursing home industry, is likely to think something like: If only we had more nonprofit homes, there wouldn't be so much thievery and so little good patient care. The image of nonprofit carries with it a halo of probity in a capitalist society: one imagines the gentle administrator of a church-owned nursing home who spends his time in good works for the benefit of his patients, rather than in calculating new ways to beat the government. Somehow the thought carries us back to a time, imagined or remembered, when there did not seem to be quite so much stealing going on around us. Such illusions die painfully.

Die they must, however, if we are to understand all the dimensions of the nursing home problem. The roughly 15 percent of American nursing homes classed as nonprofit ("not for profit" or "philanthropic" or "voluntary," in the jargon of the industry) are not significantly different from their profit-making (proprietary) brethren. Some, of course, are very good. The best home I have seen happens to have been a nonprofit institution; so was the best home visited by the young women who investigated the field for Ralph

Nader. But some of the worst homes I have seen were also nonprofit.

Walter J. McNerney, president of the Blue Cross Association, is one of those who believes in the superiority of nonprofit homes. He said in 1969 that although nonprofit institutions may sometimes be accused of professional mistakes, "you don't get accusations of kickbacks or deliberate misuse of services." However, the article in *Medical World News* that quoted McNerney went on to say:

> Yet it appears that it is not the ownership of the nursing home that makes the difference, despite a widespread impression that those run not-for-profit are better than the money-making ones. Some religious homes, like some profit-earners, are not -above shady practices. California's Blue Shield . . . found a church-operated home that was faking bills to the state to cover drugs and supplies for its private patients as well as the Medi-Cal ones. Blue Shield got a refund from the home, coupled with promises to stay honest from then on.

That same article reports on a comparative study of nursing homes made at the University of Minnesota in which the conclusion was that "there are far greater differences between good and bad non-profit homes on the one hand and between good and bad proprietaries on the other than there are between the two categories."

The term "nonprofit" does not mean what it would seem to mean: there are plenty of opportunities for profit in a nonprofit operation. All it means is that the home by law does not produce profits for tax purposes: it does not return cash dividends to its owners. A church or a fraternal order or a union or a group of individuals can set up a nonprofit entity to run a nursing home. Once having achieved nonprofit status, the home enjoys some important advantages. It does not pay income taxes, in some states it does not pay the local property tax, and in various places it is exempt from water taxes. It also enjoys official favor. The federal government and foundations prefer nonprofit operations in giving grants for special projects. In some states, health insurers like Blue Cross will only pay for care in nonprofit institutions.

Owners of proprietary homes complain about the favoritism and immunity from criticism accorded to the nonprofits. One category of complaints has to do with the nonprofits' tax advantages. Because they pay less in taxes but collect from government at the same rate, the nonprofits can pay higher salaries to their administrators, a spokesman from the Ohio Nursing Home Association said, adding that the nonprofits were actually concealing, as salary, profits larger than those earned by their proprietary rivals. Another complaint is motivated by the hypocrisy of the nonprofit designation. Like certain accusations about the clergy, it boils down to the thought that the nonprofits are human also. To me this has a faintly comic ring, for given the general level of dishonesty in the industry, what they seem to be saying about the nonprofits is, they steal just as much as we do! When I see notorious swindlers in the industry setting up nonprofit operations, I cannot help agreeing with what the proprietary operators say.

Despite the halo, it is business as usual in most nonprofit homes. A nonprofit can practice most of the kinds of swindles we have described in earlier chapters. It can engage in all the outright thefts we have described, from taking the patients' money to collecting kickbacks from the pharmacist, provided only that the gains do not show up as a profit on its books. It can pay high interest on mortgages to a Joseph Kosow. It can be the vehicle for paying excessive amounts to the previous owners, when it is bought, or to profit-making suppliers in the manner of the chain operators. Nonprofit board members often do business with the home. A nonprofit entity can be used, as we shall see in a couple of examples, to conceal excessive rentals. This was the method chosen by Harold Baumgarten, a one-time Columbia University professor, expert on nursing homes, influential adviser to the federal government.

My suspicions about the meaning of nonprofit were enhanced when Sanford Novak, the Cleveland operator introduced in the first chapter, appeared in a nonprofit operation. Profit is Novak's game, as he is the first to proclaim, and if he was going into nonprofit, I felt there must be money in it for him somewhere. Investigation proved that suspicion to be correct.

The scene is the Emmanuel Care Center, which appeared as a nonprofit home in 1971. Actually, the Emmanuel Care Center represented a new incarnation of the Acacia Care Center, a proprietary home formerly owned by Sanford Novak. It had become a philanthropic institution owned now by the Emmanuel Baptist Church, an impoverished church in Cleveland's inner city. When the church went into the health-care business, its pastor, the Reverend Sterling E. Glover, reported that the purchase price had been $2.5 million and that the center would add to the nursing home operations a family training center and would offer health services to the neighborhood.

Months before the purchase of the Acacia Care Center, the church had approached community leaders in Cleveland to solicit their endorsement of the proposal. Considerable community support was essential if the church were to receive the federal funding needed to convert the nursing home into a combination of nursing home and training center. The early proposals also called for a day-care center and a program of comprehensive family health care.

Community support was received from Cleveland's commissioner of health, the Metropolitan Health Planning Commission, and the Welfare Federation. It seems certain that these favorable reactions were due to the center's religious nonprofit sponsorship. In 1972 Emmanuel Care applied for financial assistance from the community fund and from a private foundation. The statement of purpose declared:

> This is an innovative, comprehensive, family-centered program designed to meet the unmet social, educational, economic, emotional, health, welfare, child-care, home management, etc., needs of families beset with multi-problems concomitant with existing health and welfare services that are inadequate, inaccessible, fragmented, and/or perpetuate dependency, minimum service, sub-standard existence, and futility.

It was a tall order.

At that time, under Sanford Novak's ownership, the Acacia Care Center was already mortgaged beyond the fair market value as appraised by the County Assessors. The church representatives said an independent appraiser had placed a true market value of $3 million on the business, but they would be able to buy it for $2.5 million with no down payment. These spokesmen admitted that the church had only $50,000 in cash—far less than needed as the initial working capital for a nursing home of that size.

The Cleveland Trust Company, one of the leading banking institutions in the country, was persuaded to provide refinancing so the church could buy the nursing home. One explanation for the bank's backing might lie in the church's promises of community service; banks find that supporting community projects is good local politics. However, the bank must also have considered the loan a sound one, guaranteed by federal revenue.

It was not, in any case, the first Cleveland Trust mortgage on that home. As shown in the Cuyahoga County Registry of Deeds, the bank held a first mortgage of $1.1 million and a second mortgage of $195,000 from Novak. For Emmanuel Baptist Church, the bank renegotiated the mortgage, satisfying the previous first mortgage—and encumbering the Emmanuel Care Center with a $1.5 million first mortgage.

The ownership of the Acacia Care Center then passed to the Emmanuel Baptist Church, as the license records show, although the church arranged that Sanford Novak would remain briefly as the administrator. The mortgage transactions recorded in the Registry of Deeds tell a somewhat different story. There one learns that Emmanuel mortgaged the home a second time, with a loan of $1 million from Novak himself. Cleveland Trust renegotiated its old second mortgage loan of $195,000 to Novak. The Emmanuel Care Center, although he no longer owned it, served as collateral for this mortgage— a fact that suggests that Novak retained more ownership than the official records show. Thus the church became responsible for one of Novak's debts, plus its own first mortgage with the bank and its second mortgage with Novak. The nursing home, which had been built with little or no down payment, and was purchased with no down payment at all, now served as collateral for debts totaling $2,695,000. The mortgage obligations had doubled, and the home now enjoyed the advantages of nonprofit status. As for Novak, he had turned a debt of $1.1 million owed *by* him into a debt of $1 million owed *to* him.

The Emmanuel Baptist Church's mortgage will, for the next twenty years, require monthly payments of nearly $22,000. With nearly all the patients supported by the fixed rate paid by Medicaid, it did not seem that the high monthly mortgage payments could be met except by a major cut in costs of care. The patients would pay.

The first reports on the home indicated that this was indeed the case. Complaints of poor care have been frequent, and one family has sued the home for negligence in the case of a patient who died as a result of burns suffered in his bed. Beginning two months after the church took over in

1971, inspector's reports for September, October, and November noted a staffing shortage. During the following year the Medical Review Team cited the effects of a shortage in staff: patients poorly groomed, showing signs of dehydration, and living in an environment permeated with urine odors. Subsequently, a medical consultant for the State Welfare Department and a county welfare nurse went to the home to check the medical records in an effort to find out why an abnormal number of patients, fifteen, had died in a single month. Their visit was interrupted by a fire drill. Apparently the home's personnel, panicked by the medical visit, had staged the drill to prove that they were on their toes. They proved the opposite. No one knew the evacuation plan, and a fire door fell off its hinges when a man tried to close it. This was in the home where, years earlier, Sandy Novak had proudly shown me curtains that did not come down when you yanked on them.

The most important aspect of the switch to nonprofit status was to be participation by the federal government in the training program called "The Human Service and Allied Health Assistant Training Program." The sponsors argued that understaffing and other deficiencies at the home would be corrected by the educational program for employees— but training in nursing home duties was to be provided only for those already on the payroll. This would not increase the number of employees. (Practical nurses were to be upgraded to registered nurses, although nursing homes may not grant RN certificates.)

The strangest part of the training program was that one hundred people not presently on the payroll were to be trained within what is called "The Technical and Kindred Worker track" to become vending machine mechanics, not for nursing homes, but for the American Automatic Vending Corporation. In 1970 American Automatic Vending formed a subsidiary called the American Nursing Home Consulting Company, to provide nursing homes with dietary and janitorial services, menu planning, linen supplies, drugs, furnishings, and equipment, presumably including vending machines. Its management includes people connected with purveyors of health services in the Cleveland area. Administrators of several homes complained to the state welfare department that American Automatic Vending's package deals were being pushed upon them.

One major reason to be disturbed about the connection between American Automatic Vending and nursing homes is its indirect ties with the Bally Manufacturing Company, maker of slot machines. Sam W. Klein, treasurer, director, and major stockholder in Bally has been an officer, principal stockholder, and director of the vending machine corporation. In December 1971 Bally was indicted by a federal grand jury in New Orleans for interstate transportation of gambling devices. A hint of underworld connections with Bally was to be seen in the presence until recently as the corporation's biggest stockholder of Abe Green of Springfield, New Jersey, identified by the *Wall Street Journal* as an associate of Gerardo ("Jerry") Catena, reputed New Jersey underworld leader. When Green sold his shares, the chief of the Justice Department's organized crime task force in Cleveland resigned and went to work as counselor to Bally. The counsel, William J. Tomlinson, said one of his tasks would be to help Bally avoid questionable business associations.

In summary, what had happened when Emmanuel Care became a "nonprofit" operation is this: The mortgage debt on the home was doubled, with the increased cost to be paid at the expense of patient care; the federal government was requested to put up money to train vending machine repairmen, and apparently did so, since these training programs are in progress; and Sandy Novak, the former owner, holds a $1 million mortgage.

A more intricate method of making money on nonprofit homes involves the leasing of a nursing home to a nonprofit organization. This was the method favored by two eminent personalities in the industry, both of whose images have been somewhat splattered by recent events.

Dr. Michael B. Miller of White Plains, New York, owns two nursing homes. One of these is now known as the Nursing Home and Extended Care Facility of White Plains, Inc.

The sixty-six-bed nursing home now bearing this impressive name was built as an FHA-insured project in 1963. The owner and mortgagor is the Milhar Realty Corporation, a corporation in which Dr. Michael Miller and his wife are the only stockholders. There are some inconsistencies in the various records I examined as to the total initial cost of the nursing home; however, the latest and probably most accurate figure is $779,800. A mortgage of $700,000, insured by FHA, was negotiated with the Port Chester Rye Savings Bank of Rye, New York. Dr. Miller's attorney in this transaction was Charles E. Sigiety, a former high ranking FHA official who has since listed himself as president of the Florence Nightingale Nursing Home in New York City (which was built with an FHA-insured loan of $4,068,000).

Shortly before the new nursing home opened, Dr. Miller entered into a twenty-one-year lease agreement with Milhar Realty Corporation—that is, with himself—to lease the building and operate it as a proprietary nursing home called the Miller Center for Nursing Care. In 1968, Dr. Miller decided to confer nonprofit status upon his nursing home and applied to the state for approval to sell his leasehold to a newly organized nonprofit corporation. It was at this point that I became interested, and traveled to Albany to interview state officials about this home.

The state licensing officials had some qualms about the application from the new nonprofit group. They thought they saw profit, however disguised. They saw conflict in Dr. Miller and his wife serving as administrators of the home, as owners of the home through Milhar Realty, and as members of the board of directors of the proposed nonprofit corporation. After a good deal of correspondence, however, the nonprofit organization's application was approved, but with the stipulation of a review of the decision in three years. The review in 1971 granted nonprofit status "in perpetuity."

Quite by accident I came upon a more detailed account of the reasons for the state's suspicions. An official in the licensing agency of the New York State government had been reluctant to give me the names of the board of directors of the nonprofit corporation, and resorted to reading them to me so quickly that I was unable to complete the list. On the same day I talked with people in the New York State department charged with the Medicaid payments. Here the personnel were not only cooperative but shared my concern that the high cost of Medicaid reflects dubious practices and not the true cost of providing services. It was while talking with them that a letter criticizing the Miller application for the nonprofit corporation license fell into my hands.

This letter was written by Dr. George M. Warner, director of the Bureau of Long-Term Care of the state health department. Here are some of the highlights of his analysis. The new nonprofit corporation proposed to take over the remaining fifteen years of the leasehold from Milhar Realty. The lease payments agreed to were $96,000 per year rent for the building and $24,000 per year for furnishings and equipment. The total rent, $120,000 per year, less an estimated amount for real estate taxes, resulted in a rent per bed figure of $1,606, which is 60 percent higher than the maximum rent agreed upon for Medicaid reimbursement purposes by the state health department and the nursing home association.

The director estimated the maximum cost of "luxurious" furnishings and equipment for a sixty-six-bed home at $198,000. Dr. Miller's nonprofit corporation agreed to pay Milhar Realty, for equipment already five years old, $24,000 per year for fifteen years, or $360,000. At the end of the period Milhar Realty generously agreed to sell the equipment to the nonprofit corporation for the nominal sum of $1.00—after the corporation had paid Dr. Miller, for five-year-old equipment, almost twice the most generous estimate of the equipment's original cost.

The gross annual rent of $96,000 for the land and building includes interest and mortgage amortization, taxes, and insurance. At the end of the lease term, Milhar Realty will have received a profit of $195,000 and will still own the property free and clear. The nonprofit corporation may then exercise an option to purchase for $900,000 a property that originally cost $780,000. The total profit to the Millers would then be $1,095,000—not bad at all, considering that the most the Millers themselves would have put up, with the FHA-insured mortgage, is $80,000. (Payments on the mortgage for $700,000, which provided the balance of the original cost, would have been covered by the payments under the lease.) That, of course, is in addition to their profit on the equipment. The term "nonprofit" clearly does not include the Millers' share of the deal.

The director's analysis brings out clearly that these overly generous lease payments are paid for out of patient care. The projected operating budget submitted by the Millers' nonprofit corporation with its application showed dietary costs underbudgeted by $14,000 per year. This represents about $.60 per patient-day shaved from the patients' meals. Dr. Warner estimated that the nursing service budget was deficient by 25 percent. With a nice flair for bureaucratic understatement, the director concludes that there is "little, if any, assurance of any improvements in the quality of operation of the existing facility—and [these arrangements] could increase the cost to the public." (According to a later state audit, in 1970, $154,700, or 24 percent of the home's expenditures, went to the Millers and their real estate operations.)

However, the full magnitude of the squeeze on the

patient-care budget may not have been reflected in the information available to the state. The agreement with the nonprofit corporation provided for the employment of Dr. Miller as medical director and his wife as administrator. The projected budget submitted to the state showed Dr. Miller's salary as $15,000 per year, a figure to which no one could reasonably object. However, Dr. Miller testified before the Senate Subcommittee on Long-Term Care that his actual salary was $50,000 per year.

Dr. Warner's letter of objection to the licensing of the Nursing Home and Extended Care Facility of White Plains was mailed on the very day that the official records show the change of the name of the Miller Nursing Home to that of the nonprofit group. The letter was actually received three days after the name had been changed: it was an exercise in futility. As a fitting climax, the letter was misfiled. Of course, had it not been for the accident, if it was an accident, of misfiling, I doubt that the letter would have been among the materials I was allowed to see. All parties involved—the state and Dr. Miller—were satisfied; Miller got his license, the state can show it objected. With the detailed objections arriving after the fact, the state can justify its issuing a provisional license notwithstanding Dr. Warner's disapproval.

Dr. Miller's profitable nonprofit dealings have not undermined his status as a spokesman for the industry. In December 1972 he was still appearing on television to denounce the industry's critics.* However, at about the same time he was accused by New York State auditors of engaging in one of the most commonplace swindles in the business. This is the practice of forcing families of patients on Medicaid to pay something in addition to what the government is paying. In its crudest form, it goes like this: "I'd really like to keep your mother here, but Medicaid doesn't pay enough, so unless you can help out . . ." In the

---

* On the Barbara Walters show *Not for Women Only,* telling us that the critics were doing "a great public disservice."

Miller homes, the state auditors reported, the system was more refined: in the nonprofit home the relatives made "donations," while in the other Miller home they paid "counseling" fees. According to the state, donations and counseling fees were only paid by the relatives of Medicaid patients. The amounts were considerable: the auditors said the nonprofit home collected donations exceeding $64,000 since 1969, while the other home collected $39,500 in counseling fees in 1971.

It should be noted that the charging of extra fees to relatives of Medicaid patients is virtually inevitable under present Medicaid policy. Eligibility for Medicaid is determined by the resources of the patient alone; the ability to pay of relatives, including children, is not considered. Thus the mother can be eligible for Medicaid while her son is worth millions. If the son wants the assurance that his mother will get the best of care from the nursing home but sees no reason to turn down that free government money, and if the nursing home owner can do very well with just Medicaid but sees no reason why the wealthy son should not contribute to the operator's greater prosperity—it will not take them long to strike a bargain.*

Dr. Miller's original application listed among the directors of his nonprofit corporation the name of Harold Baumgarten. At that time Baumgarten taught courses in nursing home administration at the School of Public Health of Columbia University, was the chairman of HEW's National Advisory Council on Nursing Home Administration, and a consultant to nursing homes—evidently an acknowledged expert. As an expert in nursing home administration,

---

* The industry position, as stated by the American Nursing Home Association, is that if the family wants to aid someone on welfare they should be allowed to do so. That sounds fine in theory, but in practice what happens is that the nursing home collects extra payments without giving either any extra care to the patient or any price reduction to the government. The operators are, in any event, getting rich on Medicaid even without extra payments from families.

and presumably an advocate of high quality care, Baumgarten should have been able to evaluate the Miller lease arrangement and see its impact on the patient-care budget. Why did he lend his name to the scheme? It is strange, but it is only one of such alliances made by Mr. Baumgarten.

Baumgarten is involved in at least one home in New Jersey that is set up in the same way as the Miller home in New York. The pattern is illustrated by the Cranford Nursing and Extended Care Facility in Cranford, New Jersey. This 128-bed nursing home also is an FHA-financed project (FHA project number 031-43050-PM. PM is the FHA file code for "profit motivated"). The developer and original mortgagor for the Cranford project was Cranford House, Inc. The principals of this company were David Zarin, Gerard Abraham and David Alter. David Zarin is the principal of David Zarin and Associates, a structural engineering firm, and needless to say Zarin is the architect and builder of Cranford. (He was also the developer, architect, and builder of Troy Hills Haven Nursing Home in Parsippany, New Jersey. The Troy Hills plans were used again to produce a replica in Cranford, but for an additional architectural fee of some $40,000.) Shortly prior to completion of the home, Cranford House, Inc., assigned the assets for the sum of $1.00 to Cranford House Associates, a partnership consisting of David Zarin, Gerard Abraham, and David Alter as general partners, plus a number of limited partners.

The total cost of building the Cranford home was about $1,485,000. The FHA insured a mortgage by the Union Dime Savings Bank of $1,336,000. Enter now the New Jersey Rehabilitation and Care Foundation, a nonprofit corporation whose president is Harold Baumgarten. The foundation was incorporated on July 8, 1968, and immediately entered into a ten-year lease with Cranford House Associates for the building, the equipment, and the parking lot.

The foundation took occupancy of the Cranford Nursing and Extended Care Facility on August 26, 1968, having agreed to pay in rent for the building $192,000 per year for the first three years, $204,800 per year for the next three, and $224,000 per year for the final four years of the lease. This is a total rental in ten years of $2,086,400 for the building alone—a return of almost twice the value of the mortgage in half the time the mortgage had to run. For the equipment, for which the FHA estimated replacement cost at $69,792, the foundation agreed to pay $30,000 per year, or $300,000 in total. The parking lot will bring the partners of Cranford House Associates $12,000 in each of the first three years, $13,500 for the next three, and $15,000 per year for the last four years of the lease. $136,000 for a parking lot—and that's just rent.

Under this "nonprofit" arrangement, the owners were clearing each year considerably more than their original investment.

As far as the records disclose, the licensing agency of the state of New Jersey raised no question about the Cranford deal, although the rent per bed is higher than the figure that had caused official knitting of brows in New York State. Instead, the Cranford file in the Bureau of Community Institutions in Trenton is sprinkled with "Harold" and "Tom" notes between Baumgarten and Thomas Russo, the bureau director. And not all the notes are about Cranford. In one note "Tom" suggested "Harold" might want to advise him of anything about the state's licensure program that caused problems for nursing home operators.

New Jersey did not require the filing of complete information, and could not therefore analyze the estimated budget submitted by Baumgarten. Nevertheless, the figures disclosed the same pattern, without all the details, as in New York. The estimated budget for the first year of operation filed with the state by Mr. Baumgarten is either incomplete or wrong. The figure shown for rent for the first year is $135,000 rather than the $192,000 specified in the lease, and the budget includes no mention of the rent on the equipment and the parking lot. The difference between the rent shown in the estimated budget and the actual rent the foundation was obligated to pay in the first year was $99,000. This had to come from other items in the budget, the most vulnerable of which are nursing service and food.

The same year as the Cranford deal, under an amendment to the Social Security Act passed in 1967, the Secretary of Health, Education, and Welfare was required to appoint a national council, with the function of advising state governments on the licensing of nursing home administrators. HEW assigned an employee, Charles A. ("Colonel") Cubbler, to serve as executive secretary to the council. In this position, Cubbler could influence the selection of the council's members and give direction to its activities. The department appointed Harold Baumgarten as chairman of the National Advisory Council on Nursing Home Administration, and at almost exactly the same time Colonel Cubbler was quietly added to the board of directors of the New Jersey Rehabilitation and Care Foundation, which was then about to begin operating the Cranford nursing home. These two men, one the employee of the Department of Health, Education, and Welfare, the other an appointee of the department, had found a common interest in conflict of interest. They managed nursing homes together while drawing up rules to govern the licensing of nursing home administrators. Both men publicized their appointed positions with the advisory council while passing over their business connections in silence.

Biographical information on Mr. Baumgarten was issued as handout material by HEW when he was appointed to the advisory council in 1968 and again in 1970, when the council was engaged in a series of meetings with state officials. The department listed Baumgarten only as a member of the Columbia University Senior Faculty, with no mention of his department or field of teaching. In fact, the professor taught short-term, noncredit courses in nursing home administration within the School of Public Health and Administrative Medicine. The releases cite his degree from the University of Mexico and mention some of the positions he has held. Nothing in the releases even hinted that Mr. Baumgarten was the president of a "nonprofit" organization administering a "nonprofit" home in New Jersey. A paragraph from a biographical sketch released by the Department of Health, Education, and Welfare in the spring of 1970 illustrates the oversight:

> Mr. Baumgarten's professional experience includes tenures as Assistant Administrator, Physicians and Surgeons Hospital, Portland, Oregon; Administrator, Gooding Memorial Hospital, Gooding, Idaho; Assistant and Acting Director, Hospital and Professional Relations, Blue Cross Commission of the American Hospital Association, Chicago, Illinois; and is currently a member of the Columbia University Senior Faculty.

At the time this almost unintelligible statement was released, Mr. Baumgarten was directly connected as a member of the board of directors with at least two nursing homes, positions presumably to be praised, not hidden. Perhaps Baumgarten felt constrained to veil the information. But certainly Charles Cubbler had a solid reason not to mention his connection with Cranford, since he was a federal civil servant.

Mr. Baumgarten has on other occasions acknowledged his affiliation with the Cranford nursing home. He did so in an interview with two reporters from CBS, and expressed his pleasure over the kind of people who were associated with him in it, naming Arlene Francis and Jonathan Winters. In reviewing the records on Cranford House, Troy Hills (built by the builders of Cranford), and the foundation, I find that Baumgarten had misstated the interest of Jonathan Winters and Arlene Francis, Both are investors in the profit-making corporations; Winters as a limited partner in Cranford

House Associates, Arlene Francis as a partner in Troy Hills. However, neither is in the nonprofit group. Baumgarten's name does not show up in connection with the operation of the Troy Hills home, and Arlene Francis's name appears only as a partner in that nursing home. Baumgarten's claim of association with Arlene Francis is either a pretense or an inadvertent acknowledgment of a hidden connection.

Yet nothing in records available to the public shows any financial gain to Mr. Baumgarten. We are asked to believe that the professor, an expert in nursing home administration, has, as an officer of nonprofit organizations, innocently agreed to outrageously disadvantageous leases with private entrepreneurs and is unaware that the resulting operating budgets cruelly rob patient care to pay exorbitant rents.

Baumgarten's career suffered a setback in 1972. After leaving Columbia University, he had become president of the New York College of Podiatric Medicine. He was ousted from that position on the grounds that he was flying under an academic flag to which he was not in fact entitled. According to the acting president who followed Baumgarten, the trustees held that Baumgarten's Ph.D. in hospital administration came from a British diploma mill. At last reports, Baumgarten had gone to Fort Lauderdale, Florida, to run a health-care enterprise there.

But in his day Harold Baumgarten was a significant voice in the shaping of national nursing home policy. He advised the Department of Health, Education, and Welfare on how to regulate the industry of which he was a member. Certainly it is the presence of representatives of the industry in the high councils of HEW, plus the industry's lobbying power in Washington and the fifty states, that accounts for government's continuing failure to take any meaningful action about the scandalous state of the nursing home industry.

10

Lawless Government

GOVERNMENT EMERGES as the ultimate villain. We have pointed out in the preceding chapters many examples of government indifference to patient abuse and to swindling of the taxpayer by nursing home operators. Since government has taken the responsibility for regulating nursing homes, it must ultimately be held accountable for what happens in those homes. The smell of urine in a filthy nursing home is, therefore, the smell of corrupt regulators, and the silence that answers the cries of abused and neglected patients is the silence of government indifference.

Government has failed us at all levels. At the lowest level, it is the caseworker who continues to send patients to a nursing home where she knows they will be beaten and starved, because, when Christmas rolls around, the operator will give her a fur coat. (The patient wouldn't give her a fur coat for sending him to a better home.) At the other extreme, the failure is in state and federal regulators, and the elected officials who appoint them, who refuse to hear the truth about the scandalous state of the industry because its lobbyists are shouting in their ears and contributing to their campaigns. (The patients' shouts cannot be heard because they don't make campaign contributions.)

Corruption, however, is not the whole story. It would be tempting to attribute all of government's inaction to the buying of influence, but in my experience plain indolence is equally important. The government employee, whether he is a county caseworker or a Washington bureaucrat, is under constant pressure from the operators to see things their way. He is under no pressure in the other direction. If he does his job well, he has to work harder, he faces the antagonism of the operators with whom he has to deal every day—and he gets no reward. It is easier then, even if he is not on the take, to find ways to avoid doing his job as a regulator.

One tactic used frequently is to demand impossible amounts of information before acting. If someone brings in a complaint against a nursing home, the regulator will require more evidence than the person can supply as a condition for looking into the case. This, of course, amounts to asking the other person to do the bureaucrat's job for him. This tactic was used on me in Cleveland in 1970, after I had met with a group of senior citizens who had been organized into a government-financed project to reach out to elderly people. The group had extended its contacts into a nursing home, and its members did not like what they had found. I quote from a report written, painfully, by one of these senior citizens. She is describing a patient in the Euclid Manor Nursing Home in Cleveland, certified for Medicare, which supposedly puts it in the highest category of nursing homes. She writes:

> When I reached the second floor, I had to wait for somebody to unlock the gate for me, then they told me she [the patient] was in the second room to my left. When I opened the door after knocking, to get permission to get in, I found a very frail woman crying very hard, wishing she could die. I got her quieted down a little bit and then asked her why she was unhappy. She told me how a white nurse and a colored nurse dragged her to the bathroom and threw her in the bathtub.

In one other occasion when they were giving her a bath after throwing her in, they broke her tail bone, which hurts her very much, when, sitting her in a hard chair, they tie her in that chair. The meals are very poor, she is parlized [sic] in the left arm and chronic arthritis in the hands and is unable to walk, she begged me not to tell on her as she does not want to be spit on and beaten anymore. This lady is 81 years of age and has very little company.

The delegation presented me with several similar reports of neglect and cruelty. They pleaded with me for help. They were older citizens and they were frightened. I could offer nothing more than a promise to call the director of the state health department licensure division. I was forced to admit to them that, based on previous experience, I didn't expect much to be done.

I called the director of licensure. I told him only that a delegation of senior citizens had come to my office to deliver some complaints about the Euclid Manor Nursing Home. He did not ask me to enumerate any of their complaints. Unless, he said, there is a witness other than the patient willing to sign his name to a complaint, the health department would not investigate. The health department would not even listen to the senior citizen delegation. Of course, by the very nature of the business, the only witness is the attendant who himself created the agony for the patient. Only in a most unusual situation would anyone else be around to witness a patient being "spit on and beaten" by an aide or nurse. Thus, officialdom has comfortably shielded itself from the necessity of action by requiring nearly impossible documentation of claims of cruelty.

Down in Washington, the Securities and Exchange Commission staff used exactly the same tactic to avoid conducting an investigation. The crime division of the Justice Department sent me over to the SEC when I reported some of my findings about nursing home chains. During our meeting, the SEC's special corps in the crime division left their yellow note pads discouragingly blank. They did not, they explained, have time for the nursing home industry. But they had a proposition to make to me: if I would bring them a case all prepared for legal action they then would act. Obviously I myself could not collect all the legal data of fraud; they were safe. Having transferred their responsibility to me, they no longer had to worry.

Criminal justice authorities behave in much the same way. I have already described, in Chapter 3, the mishandling of the case of Eugene Woods, and in Chapter 4, the lackadaisical "investigation" of the charges concerning Max Strauss's Riverside Nursing Home, resulting in an aborted grand jury presentation. Those were not my first experiences with lax prosecution of cases concerning the nursing home industry. Two years earlier, I had made my first investigation of nursing homes in the Cleveland area.

My data, collected from the welfare department, based on reading records and reviewing monthly journals of vendor payments, were ultimately put into a report, one that suggested areas of fraud and disclosed case histories. These histories would not provide a legal proof of fraud, that being beyond my sphere of investigation, but they did illustrate the areas in which malpractices occurred to an extent suggesting fraud; they did describe countless violations of nursing home regulations that explained the delivery of reprehensible nursing care. The report begged for official investigation. Submitted to Senator Frank Moss, it formed at his request the nucleus for an investigation by the General Accounting Office. To the extent that the GAO was authorized to investigate, it substantiated my findings. By 1967 both my general findings and the GAO report had been released to the public. But my narrative report, consisting of case histories and names of vendors and of informants, was not made public. The report released by the General Accounting Office was statistical and free of any names.

The Cleveland news media clamored for names. Ultimately the county prosecutor, goaded into action, subpoenaed me to appear before his grand jury, to which I presented
my two-hundred-page report. The whole procedure was a
rout: it was either a comedy of inefficiency or a contrived
situation aimed at protecting the nursing homes and discrediting the General Accounting Office investigation along with
me.

For my first scheduled appearance before the grand jury,
I arrived, but the jury had gone home. An unknown person
had reported that I was ill. The next time, with my appointment protected somewhat by advance notice in the news media, the jury and I met. I presented them with my report,
with the names decoded for the first time. I was the only
person in the room who had seen the report before. Nevertheless, the prosecutor settled back on the sidelines and said
in effect, "Tell your story." With no help from him, the jury
had to labor through the complicated maze of that report for
three hours. Prosecutor Corrigan never called any of my informants, never requested any of the supportive data.

The foreman of the jury, apparently finding public pressures great, eventually issued an interim report to the presiding judge. The foreman stated that he had made "detailed
investigations too numerous to relate." But he named only
one witness other than myself; the other witnesses remain
unknown, if in fact there were any others. None of the people to whom I referred in the report as sources of information said they were questioned.

One paragraph in the foreman's letter deserves quoting
because it illustrates the incredible inaccuracy of the jury's
findings:

Among those who appeared before the Grand Jury in addition to Mrs. Mendelson was Mr. William Veigel of Columbus, Administrator of Nursing Homes for Ohio, who
explained the rules, regulations and laws affecting the

operation of nursing homes in the State. He also discussed
new legislation in recent years to improve the homes. It is
quite significant that from January 1, 1965 to October, 1966,
81 nursing homes were closed in Cuyahoga County for not
conforming to standards set by the State.

The closing of eighty-one homes would indeed have been
significant, since there were only ninety-one homes in the
area. In fact, however, exactly *five* homes had gone out of
business—only one of these being closed for "not conforming to standards." Yet this absurd claim was the foreman's
answer to a two-hundred-page report detailing cases and areas of malfeasance.

    The grand jury report summarily dismissed the General
Accounting Office report and mine without subpoenaing my
records or my informants, ranging from the director of the
Aid for the Aged Office to health department personnel, and
without consultation with the General Accounting Office.
The jury neither investigated malpractices nor weighed an
indictment of any individual. They were given no case for
specific action. And that was the end result of those two investigations, the GAO's and mine.

    While government seems to sleep through the working
day, the nursing home industry vigorously pursues its interests.
We saw in Chapter 6 how Joseph Kosow made political alliances in Massachusetts. In Ohio, several years ago, I watched
a state reform effort turn into a victory for the industry. The
deaths of sixty-three patients in the Fitchville, Ohio, fire and
the nomadic escapade of Eugene Woods focused public attention on nursing homes long enough for the state legislature
to agree to reexamine its laws. On the surface, the desire of
the state was to strengthen the laws regulating nursing homes.
With a tighter code, implemented by regulations enforced by
inspectors, the appalling conditions existing in nursing homes
would be alleviated. Or that was what the public thought.

    The new bill, proposed by the administration of Governor James Rhodes and sponsored by the state health department, strongly indicated that the nursing home industry had gotten there first. That bill proposed to substitute a permanent license for the then annual license and to drop the requirement for annual inspections. The bill was sold to the legislators as an improvement.

The health department justified a permanent license on the grounds that the annual renewal procedure was a "harassment" of nursing home operators. It ignored what years of experience must surely have taught: it is easier to deny a license than it is to revoke one. Under the proposed bill, which was to become the law, a license could only be revoked, whereas formerly a license could be denied during the annual renewal.

As for mandatory inspection, the department argued that since it inspected homes anyway, a law requiring inspection was unnecessary.

I became involved in the struggle in the Ohio State Legislature over the bill, and in that struggle I learned why so many people, seeking redress for a nursing home abuse, have been denied help by a callous government. The nursing home industry is well organized, and the philanthropic homes joined the proprietary homes to fight strengthening amendments to the proposed bill. Though the philanthropic-homes gave different reasons, and the "good guys" in the proprietary groups espoused different arguments from those of the "bad guys," they were all in fundamental agreement on one point: the nursing home industry is entitled to police itself without government intervention. And the government, at great cost to its wards, the patients and the taxpayers, joined hands with the industry behind the scenes.

A friendly Ohio state senator told me that money openly passed from the industry to legislators to influence their votes on the nursing home regulatory bill. Certainly Ohio did finish with a law essentially weaker than its original law—and all in the name of progress. The department of health had worked closely with the industry in drawing up a bill which would meet the industry's approval. Any proposal to improve the protection of patients through strengthening the policing powers of the state was anathema to both the state and the industry.

The comment on money passing from the industry to the proper people is beyond my ability to prove. Yet a system of payoffs is the repeated explanation I am given of why government fails to respond to pressures to enforce its minimal regulations, to strengthen existing legislation, or even to understand the industry.

The shadow of bribery loomed once again in the spring of 1970. The Ohio State Legislature joined the rush by state legislatures to investigate abuses of Medicaid money. Despite the fact that nursing home care absorbs one-third of the total Medicaid budget, the state officials testifying before the committee at first scrupulously avoided mentioning nursing homes. Finally, forced to respond to inquiries by the legislators, the state welfare assistant director, Robert Canary, declared that the Welfare Department was totally satisfied that nothing was amiss. He even wished aloud that the other programs under Medicaid were as well administered as the nursing home program. I then testified before the committee, giving numerous examples of misappropriation of money. All my cases were documented, but all were glossed over by Mr. Canary when he was questioned about my testimony. Mr. Canary did admit that there had been no auditing of nursing home financial records and that he was aware of a few of the glaring examples I offered of the mishandling of tax dollars. He added that if mistakes were detected, the government pursued no punitive course. Both the legislators and the administration behaved uncomfortably when supplied with facts about Medicaid abuses committed by nursing home operators.

As the investigation neared its end, I met with Patrick Sweeney, a member of the committee, who told me of a call he had just had from a nursing home operator. The operator, speaking for his organization, offered Mr. Sweeney $20,000 for his assistance in raising reimbursement rates once again. Mr. Sweeney considered this an idle gesture, being convinced that the nursing homes, unable to make money, could not pay the $20,000. Mr. Sweeney was unaware of the lucrative nature of the nursing home business. He, like most people, did not realize that the owners of nursing homes include many wealthy people.

The outcome was that Governor Rhodes requested and received a 40 percent increase in the rates—a raise from $10 to $14 daily for maximum care. The following year, in 1971, the nursing homes won a vote for still another rate increase from the Ohio House of Representatives. The good news was conveyed by letter to its members by the Ohio Nursing Home Council. The letter describing how the legislature was won was punctuated with upper-case headlines beginning with OUR PREDICTION OF AN INCREASE COMES TRUE. This, however, was not achieved without WEEKS OF ANXIETY. The council reported that its lobbyist, one J. F. Farmer, had been working on the legislature for the past several weeks, and one member had been particularly helpful: MR. NETZLEY GETS THE CREDIT. State Representative Robert Netzley, who opposed "wasteful" welfare programs, nonetheless favored adequate payment to nursing homes. Netzley felt the operation had to be done quietly, so the nursing home lobbyist was SWORN TO SECRECY. The reason was that publicity about a nursing home rate increase might incite other groups to try to get more money, and after all, as the letter explained, "the goal was the money, not the publicity." In any event, they got the money and the members were advised to thank Mr. Netzley by letter.

This happy outcry indicates why the most active nursing home lobbying is in the state legislatures: that is where the Medicaid rate, the single most important fact of life in the industry, is set. But ultimate responsibility for regulating nursing homes must be considered to lie in Washington. That is where most of the money comes from; even though the states set the Medicaid rate, Washington pays from 50 to 80 percent of the bill. It was the federal government that adopted Medicaid and Medicare. And, of course, it is only in Washington that a national policy on nursing homes can be framed.

The Department of Health, Education, and Welfare, which administers Medicare and the federal share of Medicaid, is by far the most important federal agency involved with nursing homes. You would hardly know that, to listen to HEW spokesmen, for much of their effort goes to fobbing responsibility off on others—the states, the Congress, and even, on one occasion, the public. That was when then Assistant Secretary (later Secretary) Wilbur Cohen was discussing with me the department's position on proposals opposed by the industry. If the press ran enough stories critical of nursing homes (presumably indicating public interest), HEW could oppose the industry; if not, the industry's will would prevail. In reality, most action (more accurately, inaction) by HEW tends to favor the interests of the industry over those of the patients or the taxpayers. (Among many other examples in this book, we saw in Chapter 8 how HEW tiptoed away from a collision with both the nursing home and brand-name drug interests over the issue of generic drugs.)

One policy HEW consistently has followed is that of secrecy. The department has not varied over the years in its opposition to giving the public information about nursing homes; when its opposition was not overt, it was dragging its feet. In Chapter 5, we cited the time HEW evaded the intent of a congressional directive to find out who owns Medicaid-certified nursing homes. Similarly, the Medicare authorities in HEW do not feel the public is entitled to know who owns Medicare-certified homes. The peculiar reason they give is that many physicians own such homes, and would be embarrassed to have it known, since that ownership would appear to be a conflict of interest. In my own experience, I have not found many homes that are in fact owned by doctors—but if they are, and if there is a possible conflict of interest, why withhold that information from the public?

The most blatant form of secrecy practiced by HEW has to do with the reports of nursing home inspections. If there is any single piece of information to which the public should be entitled, it is the inspector's current report on a nursing home. Any member of the public should have the right to see that report before he chooses a nursing home, not to mention the taxpayers' interest in what the home is doing with their money. The only effect of hiding that information is to protect the operator who runs a bad home (and the inspector who lets him get away with it). That fig leaf was at last ripped (or so it seemed) from the industry in 1972 by the courts: a successful suit by a newsman, Mal Schechter, of the magazine *Hospital Practice,* forced HEW to grant access to Medicare inspection reports. The federal policy of secrecy on Medicare has its counterpart in the states' position concerning Medicaid inspections. Also in 1972, Michigan was forced to make public its inspection reports by a court action brought by a Detroit-based patient advocacy group, Citizens for Better Care. Other cases were under way in California and Florida.

The bureaucracies resisted stubbornly. HEW interpreted its defeat in the courts to mean only that Schechter himself could have access to the eight reports on which he had brought his suit—not that the public at large had any right to see Medicare inspection reports. In Michigan the state appealed the decision ordering Medicaid reports into the open. Then, in 1972, the Congress adopted legislation requiring HEW to make public both Medicare and Medicaid reports. That seemed to be that—but it wasn't, because, as always, it is up to the agency, not Congress, to implement the law, and HEW was far from giving up the struggle to keep the public in the dark. As of this writing, the regulations proposed by HEW would only make public an "extract" from the inspector's report, not the full report. According to Mal Schechter, an HEW official said this was because the public "wouldn't understand" the full report. Furthermore, that extract in the case of Medicare could only be seen (not ordered by mail or phone) at the local Social Security office; in the case of Medicaid, one can inspect the extract at the local welfare office. Thus a member of the public can see those "extracts"—if he is willing to find his way to the proper office no matter how far, and if (the biggest "if" of all) he happens to find out that he is entitled to the information. As of this writing, no one is broadcasting the news.

The distance between HEW's policy of secrecy and a policy of protecting the public interest can be most clearly measured by contrasting what the agency did with what it has *not* done. At no time did HEW take the simple, effective step of ordering operators of all nursing homes receiving federal money to post the latest inspection report prominently in the home, with copies available to potential applicants. That would make available to those most concerned the inspector's judgment on the home, and would also enable someone reading the posted report to contrast what the inspector said with the reality around him. That, in my opinion, is what HEW should have done long ago.

HEW's policy of secrecy seems, at times, to be directed as much against itself as against the public. The department evidently does not want to know much about nursing homes. Not only does it not want to collect information on nursing home ownership, it does not inform itself about profits—and it does not accumulate any systematic knowledge about conditions in nursing homes. (Several years ago Senator Frank Moss asked HEW to do a study of profits in the industry similar to the later study, described in Chapter 2, commissioned by my organization. HEW's response was to do nothing.) Elementary statistics—like the amount spent on ancillary services for nursing homes—are often befuddled. Apparently the facts about the industry HEW regulates are none of its business. Perhaps such facts would disturb the bureaucracy's sleep.

Much of HEW's role in overseeing the spending of its money has been in effect abdicated to the health industry. This has happened in the choice of what are called "fiscal intermediaries." When Medicaid and Medicare were created, it was obvious that they would cause a flood of paper work in the form of millions of individual bills being presented to government for payment. Existing organizations were retained by Medicare, and in some states Medicaid, to process the papers—to audit and pay the individual bills for the government. This lightened the government work load, but it also removed from government much responsibility for the newly created programs.

The organizations selected as fiscal intermediary in most parts of the country are Blue Cross and its sister organization, Blue Shield. Blue Cross is itself part of the health industry. Controlled by hospitals and doctors, it was founded to help hospitals collect their bills. It has always defended the interests of the health industry in conflicts with those who pay the bills, whether consumers or government. Nursing homes are first cousins to hospitals; their financial practices are similar, and so are the ways in which their costs are unnecessarily inflated and passed on to government. So when government chose Blue Cross as a fiscal intermediary, it was to a large extent allowing the health industry to regulate itself.

The results were soon visible. As noted in the case of California in Chapter 8, the transfer of auditing to Blue Cross greatly reduced the amount of regulation to which nursing homes (and other parts of the health industry) were subject—just at the time that much more money was being pumped into the system. In Ohio at one time Blue Cross was

almost three years behind in its auditing of nursing home
bills: for all that time, the bills were being paid without
the simplest examination of the nursing homes' claims. The
logical conclusion came when, after a number of scandals
showed that the Medicaid administration was in trouble,
HEW did the inevitable: it appointed a committee to study
the problem. The chairman of the committee was Walter
McNerny—president of the Blue Cross Association. The
industry was being asked to evaluate its own regulation of
itself.

Other insurance companies retained as fiscal intermediary have a different kind of conflict of interest. In some
states Prudential acts as a fiscal agent, but Prudential also
holds mortgages on nursing homes. It is not in Prudential's
interest to crack down on payments to nursing homes when
those payments will ultimately go to paying off Prudential's
mortgages. Traveler's also acts as a fiscal agent. As reported
in Chapter 7, the Traveler's then director of Medicare operations appeared at one time on the board of Geri-Care, the
nursing home chain linked to Joseph Kosow.

In contrast to most bureaucracies, HEW is diligent in
avoiding power, at least when it comes to regulating nursing
homes. If it had more regulatory power, it would presumably
have to use it, and that would go against the interests of the
nursing home industry. So the department has stalled, opposed, or watered down proposals intended to give it more
regulatory responsibilities. Nursing home representatives
within HEW have collaborated in that effort.

One example involves the Moss Amendments of 1967
and Harold Baumgarten, the professor-nursing home oper-
ator-consultant introduced in Chapter 9. The Moss Amendments were designed to tighten federal regulation of nursing homes, and one of them directed HEW to write standards that nursing homes would have to meet in order to
qualify for Medicaid. The content of those standards became an issue on which the nursing home lobby, led by the

American Nursing Home Association, showed its teeth. A key question was the role of the licensed practical nurse (LPN). Homes are required to have a registered nurse on duty at least forty hours a week; the issue was who should be in charge the rest of the time. Some felt it should be an LPN; the industry held that a less-trained person was adequate. It was important to the patients whether the person in charge of their care for most hours of the week had any professional training at all; it was equally important to the operators to avoid having to pay the difference between an LPN's salary and that of a less trained employee.

HEW assigned to draft the standards a three-person group headed by Frank Frantz, then at HEW and formerly with the Senate subcommittee that had written the Moss Amendments. As "consultant" to Frantz, HEW hired one Harold Smith, a former official of the Louisiana Nursing Home Association and at that crucial moment chairman of the Legislative Committee of the American Nursing Home Association. The appointment was defended by Frantz's superior, Dr. Francis Land, on the grounds that Smith was an expert and that all experts suffered some conflicts of interest.

Smith's conflict was pretty clear. He is named in the ANHA legislative news report, for June 26, 1967, reporting on the association's efforts to dilute the Moss Amendments. The report stated that:

> Because of the testimony of Mrs. Mendelson of the Cleveland, Ohio, Welfare Federation, the General Accounting Office report on Cleveland, Ohio, and on several situations in the various states, there is mounting pressure for additional federal legislation to regulate nursing homes. The staff of the Select Committee on Aging has used these unfair reports in an equally unfair way to promote the Moss Bill. . . . Because of the impression which Mrs. Mendelson's testimony and the GAO Report left on members of the House Ways and Means Committee we were forced to attempt to prove that these alleged conditions generally

were not true and not widespread. In previous legislative letters and other reports, we have discussed what was done to
combat the bad publicity. Last year, the present Chairman
of Legislative Committee (Harold Smith) and others had
several conferences with members of the staff of the Senate
Select Committee on Aging to suggest changes in the Moss
Bill. . . .

Despite the presence of Harold Smith, the Frantz group
came up with draft standards that included the requirement
that an LPN be in charge when the RN was absent. That
roused the opposition of the nursing home lobby, opposition which was quickly felt within the ranks of HEW. Dr.
Land was approached by Charles Cubbler with a proposal
that he, Cubbler, be allowed to rewrite the standards. Cubbler, as noted in Chapter 9, was an HEW employee and staff
man for the advisory council headed by Harold Baumgarten;
he was also a member of the board of directors of Baumgarten's Cranford, New Jersey, nursing home operation. With
Dr. Land's permission, Cubbler brought in Harold Smith, the
nursing home lobbyist, to rewrite the standards. In the new
version, the LPN requirement was gone, along with other
provisions that would have improved patient care at the expense of the operators' profits.

This new version, in effect written by the industry, was
brought before Baumgarten's advisory council for its approval—though the council in fact had no legal jurisdiction over the
standards. Fortunately, the attempt to get the council's approval
was blocked by a minority of council members, who were opposed to the industry's version of what the standards should be.
(Later, apparently uneasy about the whole episode, Baumgarten
twice denied that the standards had come before his council.)
In this case, the public interest won a rare victory: after another
year of internal struggle, a set of standards came out that was
close to the original Frantz version. But it took that long, and
the fight was almost lost, because industry representatives like

Harold Smith and Harold Baumgarten, and industry-con-
nected civil servants like Charles Cubbler, were permitted to
take part in the department's supposedly impartial decisions.
On May 7, 1970, Senator Frank Moss surveyed the wreck-
age of the amendments adopted twenty-nine months earlier.
Some had been diluted to the point of meaninglessness; others had been evaded. Not much was left of the original intent
of Congress. As he opened a subcommittee hearing, Senator
Moss observed to the audience:

> We say to our young people that a citizen may not choose
> which laws he will obey and which he will not. As I review
> the performance of the Department of Health, Education and
> Welfare on implementing these provisions of law designed
> for the protection of nursing home patients, the question is
> inescapable: Are government officials asserting the right to
> choose which laws they will obey? Evidence of government
> lawlessness is not lost on our young people whom we ad-
> monish about law and order.

Senator Moss's statement is a fair summary of HEW's
performance. I would add only that you do not have to be
young to be made cynical by government lawlessness.

Other agencies whose actions affect nursing homes have
a record similar to that of Health, Education, and Welfare.
We saw in Chapter 6 that the Federal Housing Administration, which insures loans for nursing home construction, is
lax enough to have insured a second loan for Joseph Kosow's associate, Dr. Frank Romano, after Romano had gone
bankrupt without paying off earlier FHA-insured loans.

The FHA also practices the standard policy of secrecy.
When I was investigating the Harold Baumgarten operation
in New Jersey (Chapter 9), I called the Newark office of
FHA to get some basic data about the mortgage FHA had
insured on the Baumgarten nursing home. The representative, then a Mr. Crowdy, refused to give out the figures,
asking: "Why *should* I tell you?" I had thought the public

was entitled to know how a government agency spent its money, but Mr. Crowdy evidently shared the HEW view that the interests of nursing home operators should prevail over those of the public. The Securities and Exchange Commission, as we noted in Chapter 7, fails to gather easily available evidence that would help protect investors from the nursing-stock hustlers.

Finally a word should be said here about the Internal Revenue Service. This book is filled with examples of nursing home operators beating the government with methods that are frequently illegal. Do they always pay their income taxes on their illicit profits? When a nursing home operator pockets the personal expense money of his patients, when he gets a Cadillac as a kickback from his pharmacist—does he report it? It seems reasonable to guess that most often he does not, yet I have heard of no income tax convictions of nursing home operators. Perhaps, if it were motivated, Internal Revenue could do what the other agencies are unwilling or unable to do—just as they were finally able to jail Al Capone for tax evasion.

Congress has shown occasional bursts of interest in the nursing home problem, although the legislature's record is good only when compared to that of the executive branch. Much of the information available on nursing home abuses was dug up by congressional committees and by the investigating arm of Congress, the General Accounting Office. In the Senate, the Subcommittee on Long-Term Care, chaired by Frank Moss, and its staff have been active in trying to dig into the nursing home mess. The Senate Finance Committee held some hearings that brought out information on nursing home financing back in 1969, when John Williams was still in the Senate; but Williams is gone now, and since his departure the committee has failed to pursue its investigations in this area with the same thoroughness.

The House has been less active than the Senate. The

Ways and Means Committee did respond to my original investigation by sending the GAO into Ohio, but it let the subject drop after that. David Pryor of Arkansas, a lonely figure in the House (he left in January 1973, after losing a Senate primary race), had persistently, and without success, sought the formation of a special House committee on nursing homes with authority to conduct a full investigation of the industry. As we have already noted, Pryor had become a crusader after he had, his identity concealed, worked as an aide in a nursing home in Washington, D.C. By the time I interviewed him in 1970, he was deeply pessimistic. He said that, after he had become known for his interest in the field, he had heard from many state and local bureaucrats who said they were prevented from doing their jobs as regulators because of the political power of the nursing home associations. They told the congressman they would lose their jobs if it were known they had been in touch with him. Pryor was also afraid to turn over to HEW letters he had received describing nursing home conditions. He explained why:

> The Social Security Administration has asked us to turn over our files to them, but I have not seen fit to do so. If I felt it would do any good I would be glad to. I think there is such a close relationship between the various levels of the bureaucracy on the local, on the state and on the Federal level— there is such a close relationship, personal and political, to the nursing home owners, to the nursing home industry and to the nursing home associations. There is such intertwinement here of people, and the relationships are so close that I think I might be jeopardizing the positions of the patients and the relatives who have written me and complained.

The General Accounting Office, as reported in earlier chapters, has conducted several productive investigations of the nursing home industry. The public has learned far more from the GAO than it has from the Department of Health,

Education, and Welfare, although the latter has far greater resources to call on. But the GAO, itself an arm of Congress, and the staffs of congressional committees operate under severe limitations. For one thing, their staffs are small compared to those of executive agencies. Secondly, they can only devote those limited resources to what Congress wants investigated, and the legislative interest in nursing homes, while greater than that of the bureaucracy, is still slight. Finally, no matter what Congress might legislate, actual enforcement is up to the executive, and those agencies, notably HEW, have made it clear over the years that enforcement is not what they intend to do.

I have spent a decade talking to bureaucrats about nursing homes, from caseworkers in small towns to state officials to agency heads in Washington. As I look back on meetings without number in a hundred anonymous offices, they all begin to look alike. (There are honorable exceptions to the following description, that is, the outraged employees who risked their jobs to give me information. But they remain only exceptions. I am writing here about the people who set the tone of government.) I am in that office with three or four bureaucrats. We are sitting around a table, and they all have yellow lined pads in front of them. I have my briefcase by my chair. I have come either to seek information or to offer it. If I seek information, there are two standard answers: what I want is "confidential" or it is "unavailable." If I am there to offer information on which they might act, there are several possible responses. Their staff is limited, so they can't look into it. If I brought them an airtight case, they could act, otherwise not. If I leave my information, months and years go by—and nothing happens. I have heard them all, and I am profoundly cynical.

It is this background of government that is indifferent to human suffering, too lazy or corrupt to obey its own laws, that makes me skeptical of all the panaceas currently being offered as solutions to the nursing home scandal.

11

New Panaceas for Old Realities

OPTIMISM IS EMBEDDED DEEP in us. For every problem there is a solution, or so most of us seem to believe. Hardly a year goes by without our being offered another quick, easy panacea to the problem of American nursing homes. I don't believe in easy solutions. A decade of probing our nursing homes has vaccinated me against any such facile optimism. The panaceas now being offered us, frequently with the best of intentions, sometimes with the worst, appear to me to be half-baked, or hypocritical, or designed to solve some other problem.

Some of these panaceas have been touched on earlier in the book. The one promoted most vigorously by the industry is that "more money buys better care." That idea should be dead by now, but it isn't. Recent history, during which nursing home costs rose faster than the general cost of living without any improvement in patient care, should have taught us that higher rates mean only higher profits. Sandy Novak was right, a decade ago, when he told me that higher rates would stay in the operators' pockets. This does not mean that nursing home rates should be lowered. If that were to happen, the patients' suffering would only increase, for just as the operators raised their profits at the patients' expense, so would they protect those profits against lower rates by saving on patient care. That is, if rates are lowered and the operator wants to keep the same profit he enjoyed last year—if only because he's forgotten how to drive any car but a Cadillac—the only way he can do it is by cutting his variable costs, and that means patient care. Nor does what I am saying here mean that first-rate patient care would not cost more than we are currently paying: it is quite possible that it might. The point is that we cannot get good patient care at any price—until the nursing home industry has been drastically reformed.

Regulation is another panacea that has been around a long time. This is offered by reformers who are as naive as they are well intentioned. When a scandal is uncovered, "There oughta be a law!" is a natural reaction. Well, there is a law; indeed, there are a lot of laws, and they have been on the books for years. Government has chosen consistently to ignore its own laws, and, just as higher rates mean only higher profits, more laws will simply produce more governmental lawlessness. Somewhat similar to the myth of regulation is that of nonprofit, but as we discovered in Chapter 9, the nonprofit nursing home can accommodate just as much human greed as its proprietary cousin.

President Nixon offered his own set of solutions back in 1971. In August of that year, speaking in the setting of the Greenbriar Nursing Home in Nashua, New Hampshire, the President set forth an eight-point program for nursing homes. This is what, in the words of the "fact sheet" accompanying his speech, the President was said to have done that day:

1. Ordered that the Federal program for training state nursing home inspectors be expanded so that an additional 2,000 inspectors will be trained over the next i8-monthperiod.
2. Announced his intention to ask the Congress to authorize

the Federal Government to assume 100% of the cost of state inspection of nursing homes to significantly enhance enforcement efforts.

3. Ordered that all activities relating to the enforcement of nursing home standards now scattered in various branches of the Department of Health, Education, and Welfare be consolidated within the Department into a single, highly efficient program. This action will place all enforcement responsibility at a single point so that a single official will be accountable for success or failure in this endeavor.

4. Announced [his] intention to request funds to enlarge the Federal enforcement program by creating 150 additional positions to enable the Federal Government to more effectively support State efforts to enforce the law and to upgrade nursing homes.

5. Directed the Department of Health, Education, and Welfare to institute short-term training of health workers who are regularly involved in furnishing services to nursing home patients so that they can meet the specific needs of the elderly.

6. Directed the Department of Health, Education, and Welfare to assist the states in establishing investigative units which will respond in a responsible and constructive way to complaints made by or on behalf of individual nursing home patients.

7. Directed the Secretary of Health, Education, and Welfare to undertake a comprehensive review of the use of long-term care facilities as well as standards and practices of nursing homes and to recommend further measures that may be needed.

8. Restated his intention that Medicare and Medicaid funds will be cut off to those nursing homes that fail to meet reasonable standards

Let us examine these proposals in some detail. The first and fifth, which propose the training of nursing home inspectors and employees, suffer from the delusion that one can train people to be better human beings. Nursing home

236 • Tender Loving Greed

inspectors do not need any more training—none at all, in fact—to recognize the sight of filth or the marks of a beating or the difference between slop and food. What inspectors do need is what no training can give them: they need to care enough about nursing home patients to put the patients' interests above their own personal and frequently financial relationships with nursing home operators. Similarly, an employee can be trained to do a specific task, but cannot be trained not to abuse patients in a home where abuse is the rule, or to care about patients when the operator himself clearly does not care. (Occasionally, one hears that nursing home operators also need more training: how do you train people not to steal?) As for points two and four, providing federal aid to inspection, the point has already been made: the problem with inspectors is not that they are too few in number but that they are too low in motivation.

Provisions three and seven are of course standard articles in any governmental announcement on any problem: make the bureaucracy more efficient, make a comprehensive survey.

The sixth of the President's proposals, for state "investigative units," has the earmarks of a cruel hoax on nursing home patients and their relatives. Known as the Ombudsman Project, it is being administered under the auspices of the National Council of Senior Citizens. Five pilot projects were said to be under way by early 1973. All but one placed power over the program within state governments; only one grant went to a private group, Citizens for Better Care of Detroit, Michigan, which had already proved its willingness to challenge the industry. Older people were to be trained in these projects to be nursing home investigators. The hoax, of course, is that the states do not need more "investigative units" to handle nursing home complaints. As in the case of inspectors, there is no shortage of state officials with whom to register complaints—there is only a desperate shortage of officials who will respond to the complaints they already get.

There is no reason to hope that any new units in state government will be any less corrupt, indolent, or callous than the existing bureaucracies. As for training older people as investigators, my experience has been that people who see a nursing home as an imminent possibility for themselves are those least able to stare the reality of nursing home conditions in the face. Even if they uncover abuse, the power to act on their findings is still in the hands of the present regulators. Furthermore, why should we ask older people to do for us what we should be doing—cleaning up our nursing homes?

The last of the President's points, cutting off funds to homes that do not meet standards, is the one that has received the most attention. In 1972 HEW pressed the states to resurvey all the 7,000 homes classified as "skilled nursing homes" and receiving Medicaid, and to recertify only those "operating within the letter and spirit of Federal law and regulations." As of early 1973, the results reported by HEW were as follows:

Homes containing 22,167 patients—about 5 percent of the Medicaid nursing home population of 450,000—had either been decertified or had withdrawn voluntarily from the program. Of these patients, only 2,330—0.5 percent of the total population—were actually to be transferred to other nursing homes. Another 17,000 patients were to remain where they were, but the homes were to be reclassified as Intermediate Care Facilities, meaning they would get a lower reimbursement rate because they did not provide the services of a skilled nursing home. The "service" most often lacking is conformity with the fire safety requirements of a skilled nursing home. The government's refusing to pay for fire protection when it is not provided is of course quite different from insisting that nursing home patients be adequately protected—a policy difference that might be recalled at the time of the next nursing home fire. For the remainder of the patients in the affected homes, about 3,000, no decision has as yet been made. Thus, of all the patients involved in the recertification, the promise of better care affected only that one in 200 who were to be moved to (presumably) better homes. Although what has happened so far is very limited in scope, it is undeniably a step in the right direction.

The Health Maintenance Organization (HMO) is a currently fashionable idea that has attracted the attention of nursing home entrepreneurs. The HMO is offered as a solution to the overuse of health care resources. Once government money started flowing into the health system, providers discovered that charging for unnecessary treatment was the quickest way to get rich; the patients did not object because the government was paying. The result was the recurring Medicaid scandals. The HMO solution (modeled on the Kaiser-Permanente plan in California) is to eliminate separate fees for separate treatments. The provider of health care is to be paid a flat annual fee for each person for whom he provides care. Since that is the provider's only fee, it is to his interest to keep his clients healthy rather than to overtreat them. The government will no longer be billed for unneeded doctor's visits, drugs, operations: that is the theory.

Nursing home operators evidently see profit potential in the HMO idea. One chain formerly known as Hallmark Homes has positioned itself nicely by changing its name to Health Maintenance Organization, Inc. Other nursing home operators have been exploring the possibility of managing HMOs (for a fee). This means that the nursing home would continue to function as it does now, but that other health services for subscribers would be on an annual premium basis. That is, members of the plan would get those other services on an annual premium payment. If they needed to go to a nursing home, that care would be financed as it is now, by Medicaid or Medicare or the patient's own resources.

The dangers in this kind of arrangement are obvious. It would be in the management's interest to put people in nursing homes for treatment that could be delivered on an outpatient basis. This is because the treatment in the nursing home would bring in more money for the operators, while the same treatment delivered outside would not, since under the HMO principle all outpatient treatment would be covered by the single annual premium. This is analogous to what happens now when a nursing home sends its patients to a hospital for treatment, at extra expense, that the nursing home should have provided as part of its regular services. Given the record of the nursing home industry, there is no reason to suppose that its members would overlook such opportunities for profit. Nor is there in the HMO concept, as presently discussed, anything that would change what actually happens inside the nursing homes.

The lesson of both the President's eight-point plan and the HMO is simply this: the nursing home problem is too fundamental to be solved by administrative gimmickry.

Keeping people out of nursing homes who do not need to be there is frequently advocated. That is an excellent idea, but no panacea. Certainly there are great numbers of people in nursing homes who do not belong there; varying estimates of the numbers were quoted in Chapter 2. They are in the homes because their presence is profitable to the owners and because no alternate arrangements exist. Some could be placed in institutions that provide less health care; there is a shortage of those institutions because they are less profitable than nursing homes. Other people could live at home, and obviously much more happily, if they were provided with home health care and other services like prepared meals ("meals on wheels"). "Day care" is a widely discussed idea: centers that would provide daytime services such as therapy and activities, and plain human companionship, to older people who live alone. It has been suggested that nursing homes could provide day care, though this is a dubious notion, since most nursing homes, as we have seen, fail to deliver activities and therapy to their own residents. Still, the goal of keeping people out of the nursing home as their residence is both humane and a saving to the taxpayer. The New York City Bureau of the Budget calculated, for example, that in 1971-1972 the city spent an average of $592 per month for people in nursing homes, compared to $110 per month for people it was helping to keep at home. And yet, even if everything possible is done to keep people out, there will still be hundreds of thousands of people who cannot be anywhere but in a nursing home. Too much attention to keeping people out, desirable as that goal is, can become an evasion of the problems of those people who will still have to be there.

Several reformist ideas are clustered under the general heading of patient rights. These ideas derive from the experience of the 1960s, when many Americans became convinced that the only sure redress for oppressed members of the society—blacks and women being two examples—was for them to be sufficiently well organized to fight for their rights. But this solution, valid as it may be for others, cannot mean anything to nursing home patients, for powerlessness is the essence of the patient's condition. People are in nursing homes because they have lost the power, physical or financial or both, to function independently, and it is because they are powerless that they are abused.

Patients already have more rights, in the abstract, than they can use. No bars keep the patient in a home where he is abused; he is a prisoner of his own helplessness. He is in theory free to leave, but he cannot because he is sick or feeble, he is old, he has no money (not even small change, if the operator is keeping the patients' personal expense money), and he has lost contact with the world outside. So he stays and accepts his abuse. No patient organization, no guarantee of legal rights, is going to change the realities of the nursing home patient's plight.

Even older people outside nursing homes have not been of much help. Senior citizen organizations have not, in my experience, been able to muster the political power and the will to combat that would make them a credible threat to nursing home profiteers and their allies in public office. Perhaps this is because older people have more reason than others to fear the operators of the institutions in which they may soon find themselves. This thought was expressed, from the other side, by Dr. Michael Miller, the White Plains operator of a profitable nonprofit home, whom we met earlier, when on the Barbara Walters show *Not For Women Only* he warned the studio audience of older people not to damn the nursing home: "You'll need it." Once again, as in the case of using older people as nursing home inspectors, we are asking the victims to solve the problems others have made for them. Older people did not make the nursing home scandal, nor did they create the tragedies of aging in America. It is criminal for the rest of us to pass the buck to them in an effort to escape our own responsibilities.

Optimists profess to see hope in the voluntary groups dedicated to nursing home reform. The organization to which I belong in Cleveland, the Federation for Community Planning (formerly the Welfare Federation), is one such group. Two others well known in the field are the Minneapolis Age and Opportunity Center, headed by Daphne H. Krause, and the Detroit Citizens for Better Care, of which Charles Chomet is executive director. Our organization has, as the contents of this book show, devoted itself to exposing the high profits and financial manipulations in the industry, though we have also handled many individual patient cases. The Minneapolis Center has made valuable exposes of nursing home conditions, while the Detroit group has defended patients and was also responsible for the suit that in 1972 ordered Michigan to grant public access to nursing home inspection records.

I am, without false modesty, proud of the work that our

organization and these others have done. We have helped
many patients, and for them our intervention has meant a
great deal. We may, in our limited areas, have somewhat discouraged the abuse of patients, though I am not so sure of that.
We have dug up and put before the public facts documenting the nursing home scandal, and it is that accomplishment,
more than any other, that gives me hope.

It is essential, however, for everyone concerned about
nursing homes—including ourselves—to recognize what we
cannot do with our present resources. We cannot change the
conditions, both human and financial, that prevail in American nursing homes and among those to whom their regulation
has been entrusted. We cannot, in any lasting way, improve
life for nursing home patients as a whole, or force operators
to be less greedy and brutal, or induce government to be less
corrupt and indifferent. The reasons the private groups cannot achieve those goals by themselves should be apparent.
We are tiny, local organizations up against a powerful industry and its official allies. Any nursing home operator worth
his Cadillac can steal more in a year than the combined budgets of the three organizations I have listed. Our political
and organizational strength is puny compared to that of the
industry even in our own communities, and when to the industry's power is added the compliance of government, it
becomes clear that we are pygmies tackling giants. Our efforts will have proved of transient value if people are led to
conclude that all they need do is wait approvingly while we
reform the nursing home industry. If that's all that happens,
nothing will happen.

I do not mean to sound pessimistic, for I believe the
goal of nursing home reform is possible if we build on what
has already been done. We have seen that bureaucracies
move when they are scared enough. Already the activities
of a handful of people have forced the beginnings of change
in government. So far, it is true, government has given us
large promises and small actions, but even that is more than

yesterday's total indifference. Now it is up to us to force government to keep those promises and to enlarge those small actions into major changes in our nursing homes. It can be done, I believe, if enough people are willing to make it be done. Individuals, of course, are powerless. To the individual, the nursing home operator says: "If you don't think this is a good nursing home, take your mother somewhere else"; and the bureaucrat says nothing at all if he can help it. But people organized in groups—relatives of nursing home patients, or just citizens who care—can make government do its job. If a few people can make government begin to move, then more people can move it a lot further. The belief that this can happen keeps me from abandoning the goal of nursing home reform.

What most needs to be done now, it seems to me, is to inform ourselves and the public about the nature of the nursing home industry, for no lasting change is possible unless we understand what we are faced with. This book was written as one step toward dispelling the general ignorance about the industry. Despite repeated exposes of the horrors of nursing home life, from Nader's Raiders to the latest news report of the death toll in a nursing home fire, very little is known about the financial and corporate structure of the industry. Government is largely responsible for this ignorance, for it has been the policy of nursing home regulators to keep themselves so ignorant that they can claim they do not have enough information to justify action —another study is needed.

Not much of what little we do know comes to us from the regulatory agencies. Most of the available information comes from the Congress, through public hearings and the reports of the General Accounting Office, or from the activities of private groups. Take, for example, the GEOMET report described in Chapter 1. That report, commissioned by our organization, demonstrated that a hypothetical hundred-bed nursing home in Cleveland just meeting all state and federal standards could provide its owner an annual pretax return of 76 percent on his initial investment, if all his patients are on Medicaid's maximum care rate. Needless to say, the industry roundly denounced the suggestion that it was making a lot of money—as it always does except when it is selling stocks —and government maintained its usual silence. Yet, aside from the 1971 report of the Connecticut Hospital Commission and a couple of small probes by the GAO, the Geomet report remains the only systematic effort to find out how profitable nursing homes really are. It should be noted that the primary federal agency in the field, the Department of Health, Education, and Welfare, has to this date provided no information on profits in the industry it supposedly regulates.

If government were forced to be serious about nursing home reform, it would set out to answer basic questions about the industry, and let the public know what it found out. Government would follow up the GEOMET report with a nationwide study of nursing home profits—and let the public compare the results with the industry-sponsored myth that its operators are all poverty stricken. Government would find out who owns American nursing homes, and tell the public whether the industry is, as it claims, made up of many small unrelated owners, or whether, as my research suggests, control of the industry is concentrated in the hands of a few people whose names seldom appear in public records. Finally, government investigators would survey the quality of life in our nursing homes and give us the information on which we can decide whether the bad ones are the exception, as the industry holds, or the rule, as the critics believe. There is no sign as this is written that the regulatory authorities intend to carry out such investigations. It will happen only when we make it happen.

So we come around finally to ourselves. It has been almost ten years since I first stepped into a nursing home. After the experience of those years, I no longer believe in easy answers. I believe only this: that we must care and we must act on that caring. "Care" in the health field is a word with a double meaning: it means to provide for the needs of the patient, but it also means to care what becomes of another human being. Caring does not come naturally to the businessmen who run nursing homes, nor to bureaucrats either; one cannot legislate caring. Why should we care? Not, I believe, for the money alone. Most of this book has been about money—the profits nursing home operators make on the tax revenues guaranteed to them by government. It is important for the public to know the facts set forth here, but that is not all of it. If it were, we could respond that, well, it's only money, and other industries are stealing from us on a vaster scale. But the nursing homes are stealing more from us—they are stealing lives, not just money. At the very heart of things, then, the message of this book is about people.

We have made the decision to entrust many of our older people—which is to say, ourselves—to nursing homes. The nursing homes have failed horribly in that trust, but the blame in a profit-making society cannot all be laid at their doors. We entrusted the protection of people in nursing homes to government, and government also has failed; yet if the government belongs to us then we share that failure with the bureaucrats. In those dank institutions where we have sent them, people are asking only this: to live out their remaining lives in decency and dignity, to die as they have lived, as human beings. That is all they are asking. And there is no one to answer—except us.

INDEX

A NOTE ABOUT THE AUTHOR

Mary Adelaide Mendelson has been a nursing home consultant to the Federation for Community Planning of Cleveland for nearly ten years. In addition, she is a member of the Nursing Home Project of the Ohio Department of Health, and of the Mayor's Commission on Aging in Cleveland. She has also served on the (Ohio) Governor's Task Force on Nursing Homes. A native of Grand Rapids, Michigan, Mrs. Mendelson holds a B.A. degree from Radcliffe and an M.A. degree in political science from the University of Michigan. She and her husband, who have two sons, live in the Greater Cleveland area.

A NOTE ON THE TYPE

This book was set in Caledonia, a Linotype face designed by W. A. Dwiggins. It belongs to the family of printing types called "modern face" by printers—a term used to mark the change in style of typeletters that occurred about 1800. It borders on the general design of Scotch Modern, but is more freely drawn than that letter.

The book was composed, printed and bound by American Book-Stratford Press, New York, N.Y. The typography and binding design are by Christine Aulicino.

(continued from front flap)

the industry and in the government agencies entrusted with its control.

- The moneylenders who charge up to 40% interest on nursing home mortgages and never lose a cent when their debtors go "bankrupt."
- The doctors who reap fortunes by secretly investing in homes and stocking them with easy-care patients ... and by making "gang visits" (the record is 90 patients in one day) charged to Medicaid and Medicare.
- The astonishing profitability of "nonprofit" and church-run nursing homes.
- How control of the industry is increasingly concentrated through interlocking ownerships in the hands of a very few people at the top.
- The incredible story of the Four Seasons Nursing Home chain, the biggest Wall Street stock fraud on criminal record—$200 million stolen from investors. For the president of the company: $10 million in pocket, a few months in jail, not a penny in fines.

This is how the nursing home swindle works on every level, from the petty corruption of social workers collecting kickbacks for committing patients who often have no need of nursing care, to such multimillion-dollar (legal) shenanigans as phony "arm's length" leases, pyramiding mortgages, ownership shuffles. This is how the use of nursing homes as chips in vast financial operations, by investors with no interest in the function of the homes themselves, has resulted in sub-slum housing and sub-human care for hundreds of thousands of patients—and the defrauding of us all.

Jacket design by Janet Halverson

Alfred A. Knopf, Publisher, *New York*

MARY ADELAIDE MENDELSON has been, since 1964, a consultant to the Federation for Community Planning of Cleveland. She is, as well, a member of the Nursing Home Project of the Ohio Department of Health and of the Mayor's Commission on Aging in Cleveland, and has served on the (Ohio) Governor's Task Force on Nursing Homes. She is one of the few private citizens ever asked to appear (testifying for four hours) before a closed session of the Ways and Means Committee of the U.S. House of Representatives. She has also testified before the U.S. Senate Subcommittee on Long-Term Care, and has submitted considerable material to the subcommittee staff. Mrs. Mendelson worked closely with former Senator John Williams (then minority chairman of the Senate Finance Committee), with former Congressman David Pryor, and with Congressman L. H. Fountain's Subcommittee on Government Operations. Other members of Congress, as well as officials of the U.S. Department of Health, Education, and Welfare and of the Ohio Departments of Health and Welfare, have acknowledged her contribution in the nursing home regulatory field. A native of Grand Rapids, Michigan, Mrs. Mendelson was graduated from Radcliffe and received her Masters degree in political science from the University of Michigan. She makes her home with her husband in the Greater Cleveland area.

FIRST ADVANCE COMMENT:
"A lively yet responsible exposé of the incredible financial manipulations that go on in the nursing home industry."

—SENATOR CHARLES PERCY

"Mrs. Mendelson has impressive credentials for this much needed undertaking. As a congressman I worked closely with her and can attest to her intimate knowledge of the nursing home industry." —FORMER CONGRESSMAN DAVID H. PRYOR

394-47597-6

PART TWO

"God save us from the reformers," Val Halamandaris.

12

Conspiracy of Silence

IN 1995 I WORKED WITH MARY AD, my mother, on her second book, *Conspiracy of Silence* (*CoS*). It was to be a cross between a memoir and an examination of the changes, or lack of changes, in long-term care since the publication of *Tender Loving Greed* (*TLG*) in 1974. She had six disjointed chapters. She had been working with someone on preparing the manuscript but he wanted to move it in an entirely different direction—an investigation into Beverly Enterprises, which was then "the largest publicly traded nursing home chain in the country." Headquartered in Fort Smith, Arkansas, he told me, it was represented by the Rose Law Firm, and specifically by Hillary Clinton along with Webster Hubbell, and Vince Foster. With the Clinton's in the White House, Webster Hubbell in jail, Vince Foster dead, and the Clinton health care fiasco, it would have been quite a story, but it would not have been Mary Ad's.

She hired me to help. Over the next two years, the manuscript grew We tried to refocus the book: we thought of it as an extended metaphor for how government deals with policy issues, not just long-term care. Although the basic story remained, we found ways to put issues into this larger and more general context.

We finished the book in January, 1997, a few months before her death: those months could easily have made a fitting chapter.

In 1996, her lawyer—the executor of her estate and also

the president of Nursing Home Advisory and Research Council (NHARC)—asked Mary Ad about <u>CoS</u>: given the breadth of its condemnation, he questioned if it was prudent to publish it. It was actually far less contentious than *TLG*, although our general conclusion was that most of the people in the "system" whose responsibility it was to protect the elderly were co-opted. (It seemed to us that *corruption*, while it was doing quite well given a $3 trillion dollar health care industry with fraud running between 14 to 25 percent*—$420 to $750 billion—per year, it was co-option that enabled it. Co-option could be as benign a thing as writing a friendly letter to a lobbyist; but when we think *corruption*, we expect to find money.)

Why the change of heart? To know Mary Ad was to know what she had written in **CoS**. The lawyer was now far more enthusiastic regarding the previous co-writer and the direction he wanted to go. But that was a direction that took the book out of Ohio, away from a host of people Mary Ad had studied for three decades, away, in fact, from Mary Ad, and away from what we feared might be clients of his law firm. To make it easier for me to represent the book for publication, we transferred the copyright to me. His reaction may also have been because he had not expected me—the black sheep of the family—to have completed **CoS**, much less make it better.

I didn't get to send out query letters with sample chapters until after her death. The 1996 Clinton-Dole campaign had put Social Security and Medicare front and center in the news day after day. Even a year and a half later, the coverage was remarkable. Of twenty-three literary agents—all of whom specialized in nonfiction, health, government, and public policy—only two responded.

---

* Malcolm Sparrow, *License to Steal*, 1996, gives a range from GAOs estimate of 14% to the low 20s for health care fraud. A 1982 House Select Committee on Aging study placed Medicaid fraud at 10 to 25 %.

One said that it was all "old hat," and everything was resolved not long after *TLG* was released. The second said that the book was "too contentious." I put the book on the shelf. Later that year, I heard from Mary Bush, the Mary Burrows of *TLG*. Perhaps, I thought, I *could* do something with *CoS*. I talked with an attorney, who advised that there should be no problems, at least as far as I could manage. Then, by coincidence, a week or two later, I received a letter from Mary Ad's lawyer saying that with her death, NHARC owned *CoS:* They did not—it was not a work-for-hire, and I held the copyright—but it was obvious that the board, none of whom had read the manuscript, was not going to stand behind *CoS*. (First Lady Betty Ford was on the board, but I felt that it was not appropriate to approach her.) The book went back on the shelf.

Mary Ad had been diagnosed with a slow growth tumor in her lung. Early in her career, she had said to me, "we keep our parents alive too long." I was nineteen and she was fifty. I remember thinking, that is easy to say when you're fifty, not seventy. But true to her beliefs, when the tumor became symptomatic, she told her doctor she wanted to be medicated for the pain, but she did not want the tumor removed. She was sent to a radiologist, and she repeated her wishes. The radiologist said, "I respect what you're asking. It is only because I am retiring in several weeks that I will sign off on your request. If I were continuing to work, I would have no choice but to insist on beginning treatment immediately. No choice."

In March, 1997, Mary Ad began respiratory therapy to reduce congestion and discomfort. Along with which, she was given oxygen for those times when she couldn't get her breath. The medical supply company delivered not the usual 5" x 30" tank, but one that stood over six feet high and was close to two feet in diameter. They would not exchange it for something smaller. After she died, the supply company did not pick the tank up. At first it was a scheduling problem, then after half a dozen calls, they simply denied ever having supplied the tank, despite the paper work and the label on the tank itself. Medicare paid for that tank either outright or through monthly billings for two years, until the condominium was sold and the new owners threw the tank into the trash.

The last two stories do not compare to the tragedies so many individuals and families suffer, but they suggest something of what it means to cite Medicare as a well run health care program.

Amidst Clinton's second term, despite the many scandals, Rwanda, NATO and UN Peacekeepers in the former Yugoslavia, al-Qaeda, and Haiti, *CoS* was "too contentious."

As I write this, the nation is discussing health care reform: ObamaCare. Now and again I hear some talk about fraud, but not the better part of a trillion dollars. We hear about end-of-life care issues, but not long-term care or nursing homes—I suppose we don't want to think about them. Some say it's too expensive to completely overhaul the system, but few say "means testing." People talk about new laws and regulations, but not of enforcement, and certainly not the stuff of *TLG*.

TLG is clearly out-of-date; but most books like it, most exposés, are always out-of-date—or so goes the argument. A lot has changed between 1974 and 2009. A lot has not.

Government is in the law writing business. After Tyco , Enron, WorldCom, and Adelphia problems Congress passed Sarbanes-Oxley. With the economic crisis, it gave us the Economic Stimulus Act of 2008 and the American Recovery and Reinvestment Act of 2009. Following the 1989 Loma Prieta earthquake in California, Congress passed a $3 billion emergency assistance bill, which if memory serves me, was reported to have contained between $1.5-2 billion in pork. In 1998, Senate Bill 927 made Lake Champlain the sixth Great Lake; then they had to unmake Lake Champlain a Great Lake. Congress passed CHIPS, the Children's Health Insurance Program, and although I don't doubt the it has done much good, and I cannot imagine opposing its goals, as a consequence of it the number of manufacturers of children's vaccines has dropped from over twenty to just three or four. Congress passed the Consumer Product Safety and Improvement Act last year: toys may not be sold unless the retailer can assert their safety (left as is, the estimate is that $3 billion in toys, jewelry, clothing etc. will have to be thrown away this year, with staggering losses to Goodwill, Salvation Army, and countless individuals who make hand-crafted toys): but "Congress provided for agency discretions," said Durbin, Pryor, Rockefeller, and Feinstein; and yet "for the agency to grant an exemption would mean using risk analysis, which is forbidden by the law. Such an interpretation 'appears to be in direct conflict with the statutory language,' Ms. Tenenbaum [CPSC Chairman] wrote" (*Wall Street Journal*, 08.12.09). The CIA report released August 24, 2009, with its attendant feeding frenzy, had been commissioned by the CIA—the CIA sent "an unredacted copy to the Senate and House Intelligence Committees in 2004, and the entire membership of both those committees was given access to the report in 2006"—but the next day, Congress is shocked. Just as with intelligence, Freddie Mac and Fannie May have Congressional oversight, so too will whatever becomes health care law.

Congress makes law. Some are good, some are bad, and all have unintended consequences. Perhaps one must acknowledge that being a Congressman is difficult.

Where Mary Ad looked at the failures of long-term care and saw first and foremost a massive failure to protect our elderly, second, unbridled fraud, then:

- a failure to collect and understand ownership information;
- a failure to see organized crime;
- a failure to actually provide reasonable reimbursement so that more honest people would enter the field and hire more and better staff;
- a failure to understand the complex weave of mortgages, loans, ownership;
- a failure to advocate for the elderly;
- a failure to enforce existing regulations;

Senator Frank Moss, Chairman of the Senate Subcommittee on Long term Care, and committee counsel Val Halamandaris, saw mostly decent and good facilities, but attributed the causes of bad homes to:*

- lack of policy;
- "State enforcement systems are ineffective", whereas "HEW [national] has done its job";
- political influence and abuse;
- nursing shortage;
- physicians failing to sever the elderly.

It is this, the Beltway mentality that shades Congressional action: problems require new laws and regulation, with lip service to enforcement. While we were working on *CoS*, Arizona was wracked by a nursing home scandal involving physical and sexual abuse. The *Arizona Republic* ran a full, multi-page, nursing home exposé that went on daily for a week. But the reporters' recommendations and the state's response: new law—not better enforcement. The state now gives a modest tax refund for families who take care of their own elderly—to encourage families to keep their elderly out of nursing facilities. While I applaud the intention to help, it fails to recognize that some 66 to 88 percent of elder abuse is by family members (with an estimated 7% of incidents reported, the estimates and definitions of elder abuse vary greatly).

But to muddy the waters a bit: while we look at Congressmen, we overlook the staff. Mary Ad wrote that "even today by their own count, there are some ten to twenty persons, all staffers, on the hill who have any knowledge of nursing homes. Worse, they have said, no Congressman knows anything about the subject . . . They determine what will be said or what will be buried."

* Senator Frank Moss, 1911-2003; Democratic Senator from Utah 1959-1977; Chairman of the Subcommittee on Long Term Care, 1965-1976. Val Halamandaris: worked with Moss 1962-1969, associate counsel to Committee on Aging 1969-1978, president National Association for Home Care & Hospice, since 1982. Causes listed in *Too Old, Too Sick, Too Bad*, 1977, by Moss and Halamandaris.

My bias is that a lot has not changed. Yes, we have sprinklers in long-term care facilities. We have better medicines and better geriatric training . . . but greed is greed, and a $3 trillion health care industry is tempting. And I don't believe, for example, that one morning organized crime said lets get out of health care.

I am re-issuing *TLG* because at this moment, the health care *debate*, such as it is with its fuss and fury seems to skirt the important issues. Will reform bring better care? Universal care? Less expensive care? What should we look for and look at? *TLG* is old. It's numbers out-of-date. People have died. But the crooks are still here. Poor care is still here. Now we are looking to expand government regulated health care to everyone, and some politicians point to Medicare as a shining example of what can be done. *TLG* is a timely warning of what happens in the shadows.

I believe, as we wrote in *CoS*, one should be a *cynical optimist*:

> While this view of government, policy, institutions, etc., is truly cynical, and there can be no answer, simple or complex, there is one path. This is the path of review and change: the truth shall set us free. Communication is vital. If information is available, reform is possible. Regulations passed, regulators hired. People arrested, tried, convicted, and jailed. The process may go too far, and deregulation may ensue. The crooks will come back, and the reformers will start over. While dubious, I hold out hope. If we understand how the process works, if we see it at work, we can make corrections and hold the wolves at bay. . . .
>
> In the following pages, it will be clear how disillusioned I have become. This happens to reformers, who start as innocent optimists. "If I could just tell the story," they say, as I said. "If . . . ." But dashed dreams, broken promises, personal attacks, threats, and long, exhausting hours take their toll. It is a process of erosion; one day you wake up and feel the gray weight of cynicism. But while I'm cynical, I'm also optimistic. The two are not mutually exclusive. To

be a pessimist is to give up. While I can't look at anything without doubting and questioning its every nuance, motive, direction, and goal, I have no choice but to keep trying: to be the cynical optimist.

To be cynical is to be aware that people are corruptible, and that the process is corrupting; that power is corrosive, and that greed is contagious; that good men do evil, and that evil men often do good. Being an optimist, in my case, is to recognize that for a miraculous summer, in 1787, the Constitutional Convention created by way of the Constitution a government that with all its faults takes into account man's fallibility. The balance of powers—a phrase taught to us as school children with such ease and facility that it loses it's meaning, like the ubiquitous George Washington chopping fruit trees and throwing his money across rivers—with its checks and balances somehow things do happen, and sometimes in spite of folly, or greed, they improve. The genius of our government, then, is that it recognizes the reasons for cynicism and it gives us reasons for optimism.

Mary Ad had worked with the Subcommittee on Long-term Care for seven years, and she thought that Senator Moss, the chairman, would write a favorable blurb for **TLG**. Instead, he and Halamandaris tried to kill the book. Ironically, if they were right about political abuse, see pages 291-293, the next chapter may show why the health care *debates* today confuse more than illuminate.*

---

* In fairness to Moss and Halamandaris, in their eight-page chapter "Political Influence and the Nursing Home," they give examples—"a *Who's Who* of New York politics," "a Texas state senator," "in Wisconsin, an office holder"—that suggest that political influence operates at the state and local, level, not at the national level.

13

"This Book Should Not be Published"

Contrary to Senator Moss and Val Halamandaris's assessment of *TLG* and their efforts to stop its publication—

> [A] pile of garbage . . . BS . . . crap . . . dishonest . . . outright lies .
> . . the worst writing on nursing homes I have ever read . . . There
> are errors in the book too numerous to mention. . . . it reaches
> conclusions that are so absurd as to be humorous . . . The nursing
> home industry will cut this thing to bits and rightly so . . . I suggest
> the possibility of a libel suit here . . . I feel strongly that the book
> should not be published . . . I shall denounce it with full vigor . . .
> [see Chapter 14]

—the book was published, unchanged. It received the George C. Polk award in 1974. Despite the critique, neither Knopf nor Mary Ad were sued. It not only received the Polk award, but numerous accolades, as did Mary Ad. In fact, Mary Ad continued to testify in Washington, and was recognized world-wide for her contributions to long-term care; and Moss did not "denounce it with full vigor."

We wrote about the letters in *CoS*, because they show just

how Congress pretends it cannot see the forest through the trees, and how it can so easily abuse its power. I could answer most points, of the type that follows—I cannot, for example, address what was said to Mary Ad by staff or about transcripts that are 45 years old. A few examples will easily illustrate the kind of misrepresentation that appears to have come so easily to Senator Moss and Val Halamandaris. Mary Ad felt that the only reasons *TLG* was published in the face of the Moss-Halamandaris attacks were that: 1) she had fought and won a prepublication law suit—the only law suit brought against the book, and that was thrown out with prejudice; 2) she had boxes and boxes of documentation that supported her "absurd" conclusions; 3) the CEO of Random House, a friend of her brother's, had personally committed to the book, had faith in it and her, and was personally offended by Moss-Halamandaris. Knopf, owned by Random House, wanted nothing to do with the book from the start.

Many of my responses come from material published after *TLG* was released—they show Mary Ad was right and Moss-Halamandaries not only wrong but show their callous disregard for the truth. But without the CEO's support, the Moss-Halamandaris attacks would have successfully killed *TLG*.

I. Political rights: Guess who has them.

I began *TLG* with a chapter, "The Shame of Nursing Home Care," that described the things I had seen that led inexorably to the conclusion that conditions relating to care in nursing homes were abhorrent. Today this book [*CoS*] must start with the same premise that quality of care is absent in far too many homes. Without that premise there is really no point to this book. . . . I had by then clearly recognized that giving the federal government some authority was not going to reform nursing homes. Only an angry public aware of the nature of the nursing home industry could affect a change; that transforming public interest could only be accomplished by a popular book. [CoS]

Several reformist ideas are clustered under the general heading of patient rights. These ideas derive from the experience of the 1960s, when many Americans became convinced that the only sure redress for oppressed members of the society—blacks and women being two examples—was for them to be sufficiently well organized to fight for their rights. But this solution, valid as it may be for others, cannot mean anything to nursing home patients, for powerlessness is the essence of the patient's condition. People are in nursing homes because they have lost the power, physical or financial or both, to function independently, and it is because they are powerless that they are abused.

Patients already have more rights, in the abstract, than they can use. No bars keep the patient in a home where he is abused; he is a prisoner of his own helplessness. He is in theory free to leave, but he cannot because he is sick or feeble, he is old, he has no money … and he has lost contact with the outside world. So he stays and accepts his abuse. No patient organization, no guarantee of legal rights, is going to change the realties of the nursing home patient's plight. [*TLG*, page 240]

Halamandaris-Moss: In response to the *TLG* quote above: *Political rights of patients meaningless—Like hell right to sue most critical.* [page 320]

Response: This is Beltway arrogance and insensitivity. It can be answered in one word, *How?*

II. George Wells: If you don't know who he is don't trust what he says.

TLG, pages 143-144:

… in a 1964 report, catalogued by the Federal Reserve Bank of Boston, on "financing nursing homes." The study, by George E. Wells, advises banks to go into nursing homes as a "sound and profitable enterprise," adding the thought that if the home takes welfare patients this acts as a "built-in stabilizer" of its income since such home have close to 100 percent occupancy rates.

Moss-Halamandaris: ***"Wells was a grad student at Rutgers, his product is not that of Federal Reserve Bank as represented here."*** [page 317]

Response: Having discredited the quote by denigrating and trivializing the author and the study, three years later, Moss-Halamandaris wrote:

Advice to Bankers… In 1964, George Wells of the Federal Reserve Bank of Boston submitted a thesis at the Stonier Graduate School of Banking conducted by the American Banker's Association. The thesis became widely circulated under the title "Financing Nursing Homes."… Wells advised his fellow bankers to invest.… [*Too Old, Too Sick, Too Bad*, by Moss-Halamandaris, page 74]

The memo listed errors: therefore this quote was at least a misrepresentation in *TLG*, but in *Too Old* it was a true representation.

III. The Foreman: The Grand Jury was "fixed," everyone is against her. Nobody listens. Her last resort is to write a book.

TLG, pages 216-218:

My data collected from the welfare department, based on reading the records … were ultimately put into a report, one that suggested areas of fraud and disclosed case histories. . . . Submitted to Senator Frank Moss, it formed at his request the nucleus of an investigation by the [GAO]. . . .

Ultimately the county prosecutor, goaded into action, subpoenaed me to appear before his grand jury, to which I presented my two-hundred-page report. The whole procedure was a rout: it was either a comedy of inefficiency or a contrived situation aimed at protecting the nursing homes and discrediting the General Accounting Office investigation along with me.

For my first scheduled appearance . . . I arrived, but the jury had gone home. An unknown person had reported that I was ill. . . . With no help from him [the prosecutor] the jury had to labor through the complicated maze of that report for three hours. Prosecutor Corrigan never called any of my informants, never requested any of the supportive data.

The foreman of the jury, apparently finding public pressures great, eventually issued an interim report to the presiding judge. The foreman stated that he had made "detailed investigations too numerous to relate." But he named only one witness other than myself . . . None of the people to whom I referred in the report as sources of information said they were questioned.

One paragraph in the foreman's letter deserves quoting . . .

Among those who appeared before the Grand Jury in addition to Mrs. Mendelson was Mr. William Veigel of Columbus, Administrator of Nursing Homes for Ohio, who explained the rules, regulations and laws affecting the operation of nursing homes in the State. He also discussed new legislation in recent years to improve homes. It is quite significant that from January 1, 1965 to October, 1966, 81 nursing homes were closed in Cuyahoga County for not conforming to standards set by the State.

Moss-Halamandaris: *". . . her study and the GAO were a rout; as evidenced by the fact that 81 homes were closed asserted jury foreman—(closed voluntarily perhaps.) Grand jury dismissed her investigation."* [page 319]

Response, continuing from *TLG* quoted above:

> The closing of eighty-one homes would indeed have been significant, since there were only ninety-one homes in the area. In fact, however, exactly five homes had gone out of business—only one of these being closed for "not conforming to standards." . . .
>
> The grand jury report summarily dismissed the [GAO] report and mine without subpoenaing my records or my informants, ranging from the director of the Aid for the Aged Office to health department personnel, and without consultation with the General Accounting Office. The jury neither investigated malpractices nor weighed an indictment of any individual. They were given no case for specific action. And that was the end result of those two investigation, the GAO's and mine.

This is typical of a number of "errors" that are either based on careless reading, or they are intentionally deceptive and misleading.

IV. Charts of Numbers: Never trust old, outdated tables, especially when the purpose is misstated.

TLG pages 15-16:

> When we requested rates paid by private patients, we found that these were frequently accompanied by a wide range of extra charges, many of which could be imposed practically at will by the administrator. [the *TLG* chart follows as shown on page 25, right column.]

Moss-Halamandaris: *". . . 1967 list . . . listed without telling of where it originated. No further, more current, or different list . . . It misstates the nature of ancillary charges which are sometimes added on to the bill of private paying patients."* [page 314]

Response: Moss-Halamandaris discredit the chart then use the same chart in their book, *Too Old,* three years later. (I have adjusted the photocopy of the Moss-Halamandaris chart by adding line spaces so the items line up.)

Too Old, Too Sick, Too Bad
Pages 86-88

On the surface, this particular home bills its patients a reasonable fee—$595.00 per month for a private room—but the "extra charges" above could quickly bankrupt an unsuspecting son, daughter or patient.

Admission Sets	$ 3.50
Air Mattress	45.00 per month
Air Worms	3.50
Alcohol	.50 per pint
Aspirator	5.00 per day or
Baby Oil	1.00
Bed Sore Care	3.00 per day
Bibs, Plastic	2.50
Bladder Irrigation Tray	1.50
Body Lotion	1.00
Catheters (Foley)	3.50
Catheterization Sets	2.00
Chest Restraints	10.00
Denture Cups	.25
Diabetic Diet	15.00 per month
Disposable Chux	.15 each
Drainage Bags and Tubing for	
Catheterization Sets	1.00
Emesis Basin	1.50
Enemas: Fleet/Oil	1.00
Foam Cushion or Ring	4.85
Guest Trays:	
Luncheon or Breakfast	1.00
Evening Meal	1.50
Hand Feeding	45.00 per month
Hand Restraints	3.00
Hypodermyclysis Set	2.00
Intravenous Set	2.00
Incontinent Care (Including Chux)	80.00 per month
Intensive Nursing Care—	
Terrace Floor	90.00 per month
Irrigation Set	1.50
Levine Tubes	2.00
Liter Cytol Urologic Irrigating Fluid	2.50 per liter
Medicated Powder	1.40
Nasal Catheters	1.00
Oxygen:	
1/4 Tank or Less	10.00
1/2 Tank	15.00
Oxygen Mask	1.00
Personal Laundry	10.00 per month
Plastic Gloves	.10
Posey Restraints	6.00
Rectal Tubes	1.00
Restraining Chair	N/C
Shampoo	1.00 per pint
Sheepskin (Synthetic)	10.00
Solutions for Clysis and I.V.'s	5.00 per bottle
Spray Deodorant	1.30
Suction Machine	25.00 per month
Suction Tube	.50
Television in Room	21.00 per room
Tissues	.25
Trapeze	15.00 per month
Tube Feeding	
Rubber Pants	
Walkers	
Wheel Chairs	per month
Senile Care	per month
Syringes	

Tender Loving Greed
Pages 15-16

FAIRFAX NURSING HOME
Additional Charges

Admission sets	$ 3.50
Air Matress	45.00 per month
Air Worms	3.50
Alcohol	.50 per pint
Aspirator	5.00 per day or use
Baby Oil	1.00
Bed sore Care	3.00 per day
Bibs, Plastic	2.50
Bladder Irrigation Tray	1.50
Body Lotion	1.00
Catheters (Foley)	3.50
Catheterization Sets	2.00
Chest Restraints	10.00
Denture Cups	.25
Diabetic Diet	15.00 per month
Disposable Chux	.15 each
Drainage bags and tubing for	
Catheterization Sets	1.00
Emesis Basin	1.50
Enemas: Fleat/Oil	1.00
Foam Cusion or ring	4.85
Guest Trays:	
Luncheon or Breakfast	1.00
Evening Meal	1.50
Hand Feeding	45.00 per month
Hand restraints	3.00
Hypodermyclysis Sets	2.00
Intravenous Sets	2.00
Incontinent Care (including Chux)	80.00 per month
Intensive Nursing Care	
Terrace Floor	90.00 per month
Irrigation Set	1.50
Levin tubes	2.00
Liter Cytol Urologic Irrigating Fluid	2.50 —1 liter
Medicated powder	1.40
Nasal Catheters	1.00
Oxygen	
1/4 tank or less	10.00
1/2 tank	15.00
Full tank	20.00
Oxygen mask	1.00
Personal laundry	10.00 per month
Plastic gloves	.10
Posey Restraints	6.00
Rectal tubes	1.00
Restraining chair	N/C
Shampoo	1.00 per pint
Sheepskin (Synthetic)	10.00
Solutions for Clysis & I.V.'s	5.00 per bottle
Spray deodorant	1.30
Suction machine	25.00 per month
Suction tube	.50
Television in room	21.00 per room
Tissues	.25
Trapeze	15.00 per month
Tube feeding	30.00
Rubber Pants	5.00
Walkers	3.00
Wheel Chairs	15.00 per month
Senile care	90.00 per month
Syringes	1.00

V. Woods: Old as the hills—only she kept up the battle.

TLG, "Chapter 3 Eugene Woods: The Unsinkable Conman" He set up residence/nursing homes. He stole what little money the elderly who had been put in his care by the state had, he neglected them, he didn't care if they suffered, he was part of having a young secretary placed in a psychiatric facility to have her silenced, and when he had to flee, he took his wards with him in a bus and then abandoned them to wander alone and dazed in a strange city.

Moss-Halamandaris: *This stuff on Woods is old as the hills, 1965 and before although she has done her best to keep it alive. The VA filed to follow up on the fine leads she provided. The Ohio Governor failed, only she kept up the battle. Is it not possible that the evidence to convict somebody (Woods) of a crime was just not there?* [page 315, see also page 304-5]

Response: One of the points in talking about Woods was to show that he was protected—unsinkable. But if Woods was old stuff in 1974—one might infer, almost benign—and if one takes Moss-Halamandaris at their word that they knew about Woods, then that suggests something.

Woods' usually housed together: elderly, mental hospital discharges, and nursing home cases who had no families, or had been abandoned by them. He protected his identity by incorporating as nonprofit, tax-exempt corporations that were branches of his own created churches, making himself a cleric in these churches. So in 1982, he elevated himself to a bishop in the Holy Orthodox Church-American Synod. The fathers of this apparently nonexistent church were listed as the operators of Villa Angela Retirement Center in Metairies, Louisiana.

Typically, he operated by opening and then closing a home only to open up another. His reasons were never clear. True, complaints would follow his ventures; but government inspectors would get just far enough to acknowledge the presence of complaints. Then, mysteriously, any punitive action and sometimes even investigations were halted. This pattern was broken in 1986 when on one night in June a series of fires were reported at Villa Angela. The firemen, appalled by flea-infested rooms, with toilets lying over on their sides, windows broken, and trash everywhere, ordered the home closed and the 45 residents relocated. The *Times-Picayune* reported the incident, and included Wood's related deeds going back to 1973.

The United States Senate Special Committee on Aging had a dossier on him, which included information from the Organized Crime division of the U.S. Justice Department. The federal department of HEW, the Louisiana Health Department, as well as that of Ohio, and subsequently Louisiana Jefferson Parish inspectors, were aware of Mr. Woods' total neglect of the elders he proclaimed to save from falling through the safety net.

Opened in 1979, the Villa was the Town and Country Motel, the former east bank headquarters of reputed organized crime figure Carlos Marcello. In 1980, he added a dinner theater to the center with that touch of drama: Woods said that the profits from the dinner theater are used to provide special activities for senior citizens residing at the retirement center, and to help offset their expenses.

Then the weeds grew, the stagnant water in the swimming pool turned green with algae; the fleas infested the bedrooms, the toilets fell off the walls, and finally, an arsonist set three different fires in one night; and the fire department closed the center, and the residents were ordered relocated.

Cited with numerous plumbing, electrical, mechanical violations, Woods agreed to corrections and the department officials returned to their offices; but Woods did nothing of the kind. He escaped across state boundaries to Columbia, Mississippi, taking his residents with him, as he had in Cleveland.

Because of complaints, the chief deputy sheriff for Marion County, Mississippi got a search warrant. He found Mr. Woods and his twenty-eight residents. Woods had purchased the grounds in 1985, converted the building to a retirement center incorporated as Church of Christ-Orthodox of which he was the bishop.

The saga cranked up again. The sheriff notified the Mississippi Department of Health whose inspectors found a number of violations of the state code for personal assistance homes, their term for Woods' type of operation. Finding no signs of abuse of the residents, the department gave him ninety days for correction and allowed the residents to remain. Since Woods had never been convicted of a felony, they reasoned they had no other course.

Within two days of the department's decision, one of the residents was found to have been missing for a week. Another two weeks passed before his decomposed body, with a hole in his head, was found a quarter of a mile from the home. An autopsy was necessary. But the body had been embalmed. The head had fallen off, or the coroner had removed it; the cause of death could not be determined.

Woods, the unsinkable conman, continued. [*CoS**]

VI. Strauss—nickels and dimes, but not crimes

TLG, "Chapter 4, Max Strauss: The Nickel and Dimer": Max Strauss was a type who knew how to squeeze every penny out of his wards. Woods was a conman with a conman's charm. Strauss was a sponge.

Moss-Halimandaris: *Interesting but more ancient history . . .*

[She asserts] Medicare and Medicaid both pay claims submitted by [Strauss] ... and convert social security checks belonging to patients to their own use ... Little evidence is offered to support either ... familiar to me because [he] surfaced in our 1965 hearings. . . 'old material'. . . Unfortunately many of the manipulations these men indulged in are not crimes." [pages 315-6, see page 304-5]

Response:

Max Strauss, the nickel-and-dimer of Chapter 4, *TLG*, deserves a footnote, since his manipulation of government is symptomatic of the thesis of this book.

When *TLG* was released, Strauss claimed it hurt him financially, but as he bemoaned his losses, he was actually assuming the operation of a 299-bed home which he named Abbey.

Almost immediately Abbey ran afoul of the health inspectors. When the numerous violations were not corrected, the health department moved to revoke his license. The county cut off his supply of Medicaid patients. Even with declining revenues, Abbey did not close. Finally, the American Civil Liberties Union, which had decided to make institutionalized patients one of its priorities for reform through court action, successfully won a federal court decision in 1978 that placed the home in medical receivership. The home continued unperturbed, giving the same poor care.

The Ohio Attorney General had one of his assistants visit Abbey. It was her conclusion that the home offered such far superior housing for its residents than they had been used to in the community that the home should not be cause of action. However, the Ohio Nursing Home Commission, a group composed of state legislators, made a surprise visit to Abbey. The legislators, shocked at what they saw, publicized that they would introduce curative legislation. Then, Concerned Relatives was informed by a nursing home operator that his brother had purchased Abbey. That made sense, since that is often the route that errant operators take when they perceive vigorous regulatory action. As the months rolled by, even the purchase seemed illusory: both Strauss and the alleged purchaser administered the home. Strauss sold Abbey in 1986.

I passed both Eugene Woods and Max Strauss off in *TLG*, saying that they represented a type of nursing home owner: hustlers dealing in petty larceny. It took the ensuing years, during which time they continued their businesses with total disregard for the regulators, to see things otherwise. They appeared to be small-time dealers by the standards then, and even more so now, and yet they had the clout to hold everyone at bay. The fact that they could evade the law raises several questions. How do they manage it? Who is behind them? How did they get the capital to start their ventures? These are basic questions that apply to the nursing home industry, with exceptions. The fact they can be asked, suggests that we cannot look at the industry as we traditionally do, and hope for improvements.

Woods and Strauss were not a type of nursing home operator; they mirror at least a good part of the industry. Even with new tools, government regulators, police, and investigators did not, or could not, touch them. But all new tools will be ineffective until we see that Woods and Strauss are representative of the industry. The pinstripe suits and less flamboyant methods camouflage the truth—the industry is crooked. That is the message of this book. Only another dimension has been added. Nursing homes are not a segment of the health care delivery system. They own more of the system than just their bricks and mortar, beds and patients, as will be shown in this book. [**CoS***]

VII. Organized Crime: keeping your eyes closed

TLG: From the beginning, the shadow of organized crime lurks, from Sandy Novak to the Woods-Marcello connection and

Joseph Kosow. This presence makes sense; it explains a lot.

Moss-Halamandaris: *In 10 years of investigation we have never uncovered a scintilla of hard evidence to support such a statement.* [page 300, see also page 313]

Response: In 1964-65, Joseph Michael Valachi, of the Vito Genovese crime family, wrote his story, 300,000 words, and

> was the first person ever to admit belonging to or openly talking about [Valachi tesitfied before McClellan's committee in 1962] a huge, tightly knit, secret criminal conspiracy in this country...[a] subculture of evil, popularly known as the Mafia until he revealed its real name, the Cosa Nostra.... Organized crime is America's biggest business...Organized crime, of course, pays no taxes, but it does pay to corrupt countless public officials at all levels, and besides its lucrative illicit rackets, it has increasingly infiltrated and taken over legitimate business...[*The Valachi Papers*, Peter Maas, 1968: G.P. Putnam's Sons, New York]

In 1966 Valachi's story was killed by political pressure. *The Valachi Papers* itself was a third-hand recounting of Valachi's actual story. If the Bureau of Narcotics, the FBI, and the Justice Department with all their resources and experience did not know, at least with any certainty of the Cosa Nostra until 1962-3 what can it mean when the Subcommittee on Long-Term Care says it has not a scintilla of evidence of organized crime?

* * *

Kosow, Woods, Bergman, and Strauss were known to the committee in 1965. That fact had puzzled me for many a years. The staff that preceded Val had told me in detail about them and their seamy methods of turning their homes into large profit making machines; of interlocking ownership; of bribery at the licensing department. They had learned these things as they were preparing for the Subcommittee hearings to be held in New York and Boston in 1965. In the case of one, they had even made a tenuous connection with the Mafia. I was troubled, however, in reading the transcripts that one man was never mentioned and the other, although named, his activities were mostly ignored. To understand the significance of these omissions, one must know something about the hearing process.

Several weeks prior to a hearing the staff moves into the city to interview key people. They line up the witnesses, prepare questions for the Senators, and sit behind the Senators during the hearings so that they can ply the Senators with additional follow up questions. The transcript of the hearings are then printed and become the source for information on the subject under investigation. The alleged purpose of the investigation is to get information that allows the Senators to present legislation based on fact.

The principal in the interlocking ownership, Bernard Bergman was not even named, let alone his business connections. In the hearing where organized crime had surfaced, one such connection, Joe Kosow, was mentioned once, with no hint of his shady connections. No one asked any follow up questions to the witness who mentioned him; nothing about interlocking ownership, trafficking in homes, usurious rates charged by an SBA, not even on the number of homes owned directly or indirectly by these men and their relationships to business peripheral to their nursing homes. I knew of these men and these subjects because the staff for the Senators—the same Senators who did not ask the questions—had told me. [*CoS**]

Legally, there is only evidence if a it has been admitted into a judicial or legislative investigation. If witnesses aren't called or good, probing, thoughtful, cogent questions asked—questions aimed at digging into a situation and determining the who, what, where, why, when and how of things—there is no evidence, *not a scintilla*.

* * *

In 1977, Val was the drawing card for National Citizens Co-alition for Nursing Home Reform. He began with a story that left many of the audience confused

A man, Mr. X, completed his prison sentence for forging checks and got a job as the administrator in a California nursing home. He worked hard at his job, by that he meant that he wined and dined the right people at a mental health hospital in order to keep his home at 135 percent occupancy. Inspectors overlooked this violation because he had political protection from a well placed person who had an interest in the home.

Mr. X and the owner, Harry, also had a "board and care home" next door. Its expenses were passed on to Medicaid through the nursing home since board and care homes cannot be supported by Medicaid. This pass through, too, was overlooked.

The two homes served as the genesis for cash which flowed into a secret fund. One day, Mr. X drew money from this fund for a trip to Las Vegas. When returned, he learned that Harry had been subpoenaed to testify at a grand jury investigation. In describing the grand jury incident, Val stressed that Harry had been provided with all of the questions that he would be asked so that he would have the right answers: clearly Harry had connections.

Mr. X became frightened, and approached a state Senator whose response was enigmatic. However, Mr. X understood; Harry had powerful friends. The Senator dared not to get entangled.

Mr. X went to an assistant attorney general. Val pointed to me, seated in the back of the auditorium, and said that the assistant attorney general had just read *TLG*. As a result, he had decided that he should investigate the nursing home industry. Mr. X's story intrigued him. He said he would investigate.

Shortly after this meeting, Mr. X taped an admission from the owner that he had been provided with the questions prior to testifying and that he had been protected from an indictment. One day, the administrator, Mr. X, was driving home when a car pulled along side, and Val imitated a machine gun: the administrator was shot.

Mr. X was hospitalized with a nervous breakdown as well as for his gunshot wounds. His wife left him. The Attorney General quashed the investigation. When Mr. X left the hospital, he went to Val at the U.S. Senate Special Committee on Aging. Val vowed to act.

Then he asked us, was this the Mafia? [*CoS**]

* * *

In early 1978, Jack Anderson wrote that there was disturbing evidence that the "mob" was siphoning off federal money. Mr. Anderson described in some detail the testimony of one witness, an unnamed psychiatrist, before a federal grand jury in 1976. He told the prosecutors that crime lords had ways of taking hundreds of thousands of dollars from the federal health programs. A member of the Vito Genovese crime family was a silent partner in a Bronx welfare clinic. Twenty to twenty-five percent of the clinic's income went to him. The doctor, himself, had to make monthly payments to an associate of the partner just to practice psychiatry. The doctor also said that the mob threatened owners of Medicaid clinics with beating and arson if they did not pay the mob. In return, the mob promised political assistance and protection from competition. These payoffs were concealed in inflated charges.

Another paragraph in the Anderson story mirrored the previous chapter in this book [*CoS*], on the maze of ownership. He wrote that the crime connections hide behind a murky curtain of legitimate enterprises, dummy corporations and holding companies. Notorious mobsters like Meyer Lansky, Joe Columbo reportedly have been linked to nursing homes, hospitals, and clinical laboratories, although their ownership has been obscured by this corporate web. [*CoS**]

* * *

In August, 1996, Stefano Mazzola, who served time for armed robbery and loansharking was charged with bribing people to bring new members to his HMOs or preferred provider organizations associated with New Jersey based Tri-Con Associates, of which he was chief economic officer. It is alleged he made money for the mob through bribery and extortion. Investigators taped hundreds of conversations with alleged members of the Genovese crime family, reputedly led by Vincent "The Chin" Gigante of New York. The director of the state Division of Criminal Justice said that he thought they would prove that there was involvement at that upper level. New Jersey Attorney General Peter Verniero said: "We are alleging for the first time the involvement of organized crime in the health care industry."

"For the first time." I am reminded of Senator Moss's 1974 comment that ten years of investigation had failed to disclose a scintilla of evidence of the presence of organized crime. [*CoS**]

* * *

Dr. W_____ was the number two man in the Department of Health. He was convinced that organized crime, which he referred to as the Mafia, owned nursing homes. One of the reasons for his conclusion was that too many things are omitted. In his mind, omissions were as damning as the actual use of names known to be members of the Mafia.

Dr. W_____ had grown up in a neighborhood with a Mafia family. He had watched the first generation send their sons to Harvard and Yale. He then saw them become bankers and lawyers which are ideal positions to further the Mafia interest in land deals, in financing, and in construction.

He saw construction as an exceedingly important part of the Mafia connection. And, indeed, many a nursing home chain has its own construction company. He believed that the nursing home applicant for a Certificate of Need [referring to a specific home] submitted costs of building that far exceeded the real cost. The inflated cost of construction then becomes the base of the cost of ownership item in determining government reimbursement.

He found the financing of nursing homes strange. Since the industry is financially successful, he argued that there should be foreign investors because that money flows into money making businesses. The absence of such names has an ominous ring to it.

Dr. W_____ became curious about the Medicaid rates. The state Department of Human Services, did not share the Medicaid rates with the Health Department. He was, however, able to get some of the material. He found it shocking. The range of variation in rates was inexplicable. Why, he asked, should one 50-bed home get ten dollars more a day per Medicaid patient than another? The constant barrage of unanswerable questions helped to convince him that organized crime was the explanation.

Dr. W_____ spoke freely of people in his department, in the welfare department, and in the regional office of HHS who were paid off to overlook discrepancies. He also knew that there were civil servants who were simply frightened. They were not corrupt, but they did allow the industry to operate with greased wheels. The things that he told me reinforced my own findings, but they came from a man second in command of the department that oversees the medical needs of patients. One point he made is highly significant: the absence of action or omissions are as important as the actual name of a known member of the crime world. There is a plethora of unexplained inaction and of omission in the nursing home industry.

The most serious inactivity, as far as permitting unnecessarily high health costs, is the inattention paid to fraud. I've mentioned some of the government programs which almost imme-

diately flounder as if by design. Because so little is actually done
by government against nursing home operators, there is no supportive data to prove the extent of fraud. Not even HHS, divided
as it is into regional offices with personnel assigned to each state,
has a data bank on the activities of state investigations or media
stories. The absence of information, combined with the stricter
laws to control fraud, which have not been used, underscore Dr.
W_____'s contention that these are in reality signs of the presence of organized crime.

I interviewed Dr. W_____ several times. While he was forth-
right with me, he said, with trembling hands, "Please respect the
confidentiality of our interview. If people found out, they will kill
me." Dr. W_____ died a few years ago. [*CoS**]

VIII. Bergman: Old stuff going back fifteen years, and perfect-ly legal.

When Knopf sent Moss the galleys in 1973, Mary Ad was
no stranger to the Committee on Aging or the Subcommittee on
Long-Term Care—she had worked with them since 1966. *TLG*
described the "ancient history" of Dr. Bergman's ownership,
mortgage, and loan scams, which, Moss said was known to the
Senate Subcommittee on Long-term Care, Senator Moss, and Val
Halamandaris as early as 1959.

In their letters to Knopf, Moss and Halamandaris tried to
discredit *TLG* by trivializing and dismissing Mary Ad's discus-
sion of Dr. Bernard Bergman:

> ... Dr. Bergman ... [is] familiar to me because ... [he] surfaced
> in our 1965 hearings. I agree with Elliot Richardson that much of
> what she has is "old material" (page 125) going back as far as 1959,
> 1960 and 1962. . . . The author provides little that we did not have

in 1965. Unfortunately many of the manipulations these men indulged in **are not crimes** . . . I deplore an effort in this book to tie in extraneous data much of it misused or false to create inferences or conclusions . . . More ancient history on our friend Dr. Bergman 1965, 66 and 68. They [Mary Ad & David Hapgood] really miss the point in this chapter. They blast HEW for not enforcing Moss amendment requiring that those with 10 percent interest in nursing homes disclose such interest. States now comply. **HEW has done its job**. . . . They are off base when they say ownership is hidden so as to facilitate a sale and lease back arrangement. . . [which] is **perfectly legal** tax device used openly by the best of companies. [emphasis added; pages 304-5, 316-7]

The Senator's overall position can be restated: *evidence for what Mendelson says is at best scant, and what there is, is old, misleading or dishonest, for example: Dr. Bergman.*

And yet:

In the summer of **1974**, the city of New York **virtually exploded** in the wake of a newspaper exposé about nursing homes written by *New York Times* writer John Hess. . . . [Following] an audit of the 347-bed Towers Nursing Home owned by Rabbi **Bernard Bergman**. . . . [Which] set off **more shock waves**. . . . . Mr. Bergman, who in a short time had built himself a $24million nursing home and a related real estate empire largely out of Medicaid funds. What made the Bergman case unique was not the many allegations of poor care and abuse nor the fact that $2.2 million could not be accounted for . . . [it] was the revelation of the involvement of New York's major political figures with nursing homes. . . . most of the nation [was] **shocked** to learn of the extent to which politicians used their influence to benefit nursing home interests. [*Too Old*, page 163; emphasis added]

So wrote Senator Moss and Val Halamandaris just three years later in their 1977 *Too Old Too Sick Too Bad: Nursing Homes*

in America: three years after asserting to Knopf—and others—
that Bergman was "ancient history," and what he was doing was,
by way of two attorneys general, "perfectly legal." No mention of
their apparent failure to understand the nature and extent Bergman's crimes, no mention of Mary Ad's warnings: but following
the news stories and the audit, following the release of *TLG*,
the Subcommittee on Long-Term Care proudly investigated Dr.
Bergman—just as all the committees and subcommittees in the
House and the Senate are investigating the regulatory failures that
led to the 2008-2009 financial and economic disaster today.

The only reference to Bergman in their 326 page book, is
Chapter 11, "Political Influence and the Nursing Home," pages
163-170, devoted to Rabbi Bergman's local and state political
connections:

> . . . most of the nation was shocked to learn of the extent to which
> politicians used their influence to benefit nursing home interest . .
> . another type of abuse of political power is obtaining preferences
> for nursing home operators . . . bogus hearings . . . to complete
> the "white wash," elected officials have issued reports proclaiming
> their state free from any serious nursing home problems . . . Still
> other abuses involve legislators . . . the Moreland Commission re-
> port . . . reads like a novel of political intrigue . . .

But Bergman "asserted his constitutional rights against self-
incrimination"—or as *Time* wrote February 3, 1975, "The committee produced little solid evidence against Bergman." So "it
remained for New York's Moreland Act commission on Nursing
Home and Residential facilities to complete the probe into *political influence and related issues*" (*Too Old,* 164; emphasis added).

Despite saying "$24 million nursing home and a related real
estate empire" or "allegations of poor care," one would little guess
the extent of that empire, or the great harm Bergman committed to hundreds of elderly patients, from their book: one might

presume that the well informed senator, counsel and committee, while "deploring" Bergman's actions, concurred with Attorneys General Richardson and Brooke: some of those actions were "perfectly legal." After all their greatest concern, the subject of the chapter, was "New York . . . political influence."

On the face of it, when they wrote their letters, they didn't know about the extent of Bergman's political connections (the findings of the Moreland Commission), nor did they know the full extent of Bergman's complex ownership interests in nursing homes, real estate, buildings and companies, from Florida to New York, and inland to Ohio, Illinois, and Colorado (the result of investigations in New York): So what did they mean by "old material" and "ancient history"?

Perhaps they did know these things—the state investigation had begun well before their letters to Knopf; would not state investigators have talked with the Subcommittee, and if not, why?—and were themselves committing a "type of abuse of political power."

In 1976, Bergman was sentenced to jail on Federal and state charges that included Medicare, Medicaid and tax fraud ("perfectly legal"?)—and ordered to repay $2 million.

What of the "patients . . . brought to the emergency room in a coma from dehydration . . bed sores . . . serious diarrhea epidemic . . . excrement on the floors," (*Time*, 02.03.75)? Where Mary Ad despaired at elderly patients' lack of power, political, legal, and medical—powerless to prevent life threatening dehydration, bed sores, malnutrition, theft, physical and sexual assault—Halamandaris arrogantly said, "Political rights of patients meaningless [from *TLG*]—Like hell right to sue most critical" (page 320). Of the thousands of patients that found themselves in Rabbi Bergman's tender loving care, how many did or could have exercised that right? (Before getting that far, if someone could, *troublesome* patients were often transferred to psychiatric facilities or reported as having psychiatric problems (for example, see ***TLG*** pages 67-71): rendering their testimony virtually unusable.) How many may simply have died first?

The following chart, "Nursing Home Interlocking Ownership and Interests, 12/31/73 . . . Network Analysis/Chart by Kal Lee, NYC" was part of the evidence developed against Bergman by officials in New York. Every The charts shows nursing homes, and real estate, holding and related companies in which he had full or partial ownership. The connecting lines show how the companies are related. The chart is not complete.

NURSING HOME INTERLOCKING OWNERSHIP

[This facsimile is difficult to read in the original 2'x3', and is not defective in printing.]

NETWORK ANALYSIS/CHART BY HAL LEE - NYC

[This facsimile is difficult to read in the original 2'x3', and is not defective in printing.]

14

The Letters

Here is the text of the December 5, 1973, letter from Senator Frank Moss, Chairman, Subcommittee on Long-Term Care to David Bain, assistant to Regina Ryan, editor of *TLG*, at Knopf (emphasis in the original). The letter included an enclosure, probably the Halamandaris memo, but there is no way to know for certain.

Dear Mr. Bain:

Thank you and Mrs. Ryan for an opportunity to comment on the proposed books *Tender Loving Greed,* by Mary Adelaide Mendelson. I appreciate the kind words about me and the work of my Subcommittee on Long-Term Care. I sincerely wish that I could tell you that this manuscript is accurate, constructive and an intelligent contribution to the battle we have been waging to improve life for the one million Americans who suffer the compound burdens of illness and advanced age.

In fact, the book is far from accurate. There are errors in the book too numerous to mention. Facts are few and far between. Inferences and generalizations abound. It gives currency to rumors that are sometimes outright lies. Piling inference on top of inference it reaches conclusions that are so absurd as to be humorous. In short, it lacks integrity and for this reason it is a very destructive writing. I don't know when I have been more disappointed and distressed. Here are a few examples of what I mean:

1. Inaccurate Generalizations

From the very beginning the book asserts the nursing home *industry* is exploiting the poor and defrauding all of us. There is no room left for doubt that the author's criticism is leveled at each and every operator in the U.S. These charges are made on pages 24, 340 299 48, 129, 155. On page 30 the author states, "It disturbs me that I seem to be indicting all nursing homes in one sweep of the brush." She goes on to say that she has been in 200 homes and only seen one good one. On page 157, she notes that non-profit homes are "not significantly different from profit homes." The Book, [sic] in short, is a blanket indictment of an entire industry.

Comment: This is a blatantly false premise that runs through the entire book. *All* nursing home operators are not dishonest any more than *all* politicians are on-the take. Applying another analogy, it is like saying that all Italians are members of the Mafia. More such hasty generalizations follow.

-2-

• It is alleged (as noted above) that all operators are making "incredible profits" (p.48, 34, 24, 129, 155), that there is "thievery and corruption in our stinking nursing homes."

Comment: Our studies show that it is almost impossible to generalize about nursing home profits. Some operators are making large profits and some are going broke. Goals and expectations differ. Operators set different goals, some seek to maximize equity, some seek to minimize equity. Some seek high profits before taxes, others seek after tax profits. Some actively seek tax loses with which to offset taxable gains in other business. Just as these expectations differ, their ability to reach these expectations differ. The results of our studies will be made public soon. The Department of HEW is undertaking a separate study (contrary to what was said on P.180) of nursing home profits and costs. The results of this study show that there is not much difference in cost across the nation between the average for a skilled nursing home and an intermediate care facility (less than a dollar per day per on the average). This is contrary to the author's statement (top of page 43) that intermediate care facilities "cost . . . a little more than half . . . that of a skilled nursing home."

P.17, "Cadillacs are standard equipment for this business"— asserting that all nursing home operators drive Cadillacs as a result of high profits. Assertion repeated P.34, 35, 106, 183, 186.

Comment: This is a ridiculous and untrue conclusion.

• Paraphrasing:"TheMafiaisinvolvedinnursinghomes,"p.17,65,163.

Comment: In 10 years of investigation we have never uncovered a scintilla of hard evidence to support such a statement. This the author admits on page 88, but the inferences in other sections of the book are allowed to stand.

• The statement is made on page 18, that there is no relationship between the dollars paid and the quality of care. See also pages 29, 36, 155.

Comment: This is false. The reimbursement system and the amount of money States pay for welfare patients is the most important factor in the quality of care according to a study by Dr. Nancy Anderson, University of Minnesota, cited by the authors in a different context on page 159.

• On page 29 the author states that "regulations make no difference" and that nursing homes are similar everywhere and "similarly bad" in every State of the Union.

Comment: The conclusion is patently ridiculous. There are great differences in the quality of care offered in various States in the Union. Regulations and the vigor of State enforcement policies differ. Connecticut requires one registered nurse for every 30 patients on the day shift, one for every 45 on the afternoon shift and one for every 60 on the night shift. The Federal standard is only one RN on the 7 a.m. to 3 p.m. shift and the minimum of a LPN in charge on the other

-3-

two shifts. Many States do not even meet these Federal minimums.

The quality of care in Mississippi, Pennsylvania and Massachusetts is far different from Connecticut.

• On page 18 another recurrent theme occurs, that *all* providers charge for non-delivered services. The assertion is repeated in many places throughout Chapter 8.

Comment: All providers (suppliers would be a better word) do not seek to defraud the government. Contrary to the assertion in Chapter 8 that cases involving "Ancillary charges" are the most well documented examples of fraud and corruption, I have seen little evidence of abuse concerning morticians, linen suppliers, or ambulance drivers. I have seen precious little on physicians. What evidence there is relates to drug kickbacks. Even there the evidence is contradictory. The good evidence that is available is not cited in the book. There is no new evidence on the activities of any other suppliers. On page 151, there is a reference to the fact that 35 doctors collected $3 million from Medicaid and that eleven dentists collected $1 million. The reference is oblique, implying that this happened in nursing homes. My instincts tell me that the citation refers to the Medicaid program in general of which nursing homes are a small part.

The few references to physicians' "gang visits" are accurate but we feel this is not a significant problem in view of the IRS corrective action. IRS action was apparently missed by the author who blasts them for non-action on page 183. IRS automatically audits the returns of physicians with incomes over $25,000 who have substantial claims coming from Medicare and Medicaid. Medicare, and Medicaid send duplicate vouchers with the physician number to IRS. We have found that the bigger problem is to get doctors to go to nursing homes rather than in doctors providing care that isn't needed.

• The author states on page 157, that there is very little difference between non-profit and for profit homes, implying that both are bad.

Comment: It is certainly true that some homes use non-profit status as a guise. It is also true that most do not. In my experience, the best homes in the U.S. are church owned, related and operated and therefore non-profit. I am not willing to concede that there are no differences between for-profit and non-profit homes. There are some significant studies which show more staff in non-profit homes, higher salaries for employees and lower turnover rates for aides and employees. Against this, the author offers one Minnesota study and two examples. Chapter 9 is extremely weak.

2. *A few Obvious Errors*

A. The author's use of General Accounting Office audits is extremely casual. A few examples:

Page 32 "GAO turned up *swindles* in six other States," among them Oklahoma, Michigan, and New York. This is an obvious reference to the May 28, 1971 audit

-4-

of these three States. The audit measures whether fire safety, physicians and nursing standards were being met and points out a lack of a uniform definition of skilled nursing care in the 50 states.

On page 42 the author uses this same report to argue that many people are in nursing homes who don't belong there. "GAO concluded . . . that 80 percent of the patients in Michigan did not need nursing care."

Comment: GAO stated that when one set of criteria was applied 42 percent of he patients in Michigan did not need *skilled* nursing care. When another set of criteria were applied 79 percent did not need *skilled* nursing care. It did not say that they did not need nursing home care, just that there was no uniform definition and that some people needed a *different level of* nursing home care.

• Page 32, the author asserts that GAO is doing a study of profits in Oregon and Florida.

Comment: GAO and the Committee staff completed a study of Tennessee, Massachusetts and Colorado for our forthcoming report. There is no study of Oregon and Florida according to my information.

• Page 36, there is an assertion that GAO has undertaken a study showing nursing homes with a 450 percent return on investment in five years.

Comment: There is no such study according to my information.

B. The Invocation of the Subcommittee Name

The name of the Subcommittee on Long-Term Care is used on several occasions. Attributions are made to the Subcommittee and its staff which should not be made. On page 105, 124, 125, and 126, it is asserted that the Subcommittee presented information with respect to Mr. Kosow to the then Attorney General of Massachusetts, Edward Brooke. The book charges that the Attorney General did not conduct a vigorous investigation. This charge is attributed to me rather than the author, e.g. "The Subcommittee thought that the answer might lie in campaign contributions (to the Brooke-for-Senator campaign)."

Comment: The Subcommittee is made up of myself and 16 other members of the Senate (1965). I have never leveled such a charge and to the best of my recollection neither did any other member of the Committee. I doubt any member of the staff made any such statement. Moreover, the staff members are without authority to make such a charge. To this day I respect Senator Brooke's statement to me that he was "not in possession of sufficient probative facts to state that these irregular and questionable actions were of criminal nature."

C. Other Errors

• On page 147 the book uses a quote from an unnamed persons (Ellen Marx)

-5-

who appeared at our Minnesota hearings. This witness was greatly discredited in follow-up hearings held by the State.

• Mrs. Daphne Krause did not testify that 25 percent of nursing homes have drug problems. She said about 25-30 percent of the homes in Minnesota had serious abuses some of which were drug problems.

• On page 145 the author misquotes Associate Counsel Val J. Halamandaris Senate Special Committee on Aging. He stated that 40 percent of nursing home drugs were classified as *central nervous system drugs.* The author's language suggested counsel said that 40 percent of drugs were either tranquilizers or sedatives. This is not true. To be exact 19 percent are tranquilizers, about 10 percent are sedatives and another 10 percent are analgesics, including drugs like Darvon and aspirin.

This brings up another error, page 146 which charges nursing homes supply a prescription drug (darvon [sic]) instead of an aspirin because the latter should be furnished as part of the homes general supplies. This is untrue. Both drugs are paid for by Medicaid if prescribed by a doctor (even in the State of Ohio) according to the GAO study for the Committee which Mr. Halamandaris cites.

• Pages 159 and 170, Harold Baumgarten is charged with great influence on government nursing home policy. In reality, he had little. Some of the little influence he had might have even been constructive. For example, his Committee recommended in strong language that Nursing Home Licensure Boards set up by the states should not be dominated by the nursing home industry. Moreover, I am informed that he is in Denver and not Florida.

With respect to Dr. Miller in the same chapter, I am informed that the State of New York did have problems with the quality of care in the early days but that care is adequate to good at the present times. I have seen no proof that he subsidized Medicaid in violation of the law. I suggest the possibility of a libel suit here.

• Senator Russell Long assures me that he has no nephew serving as counsel or in any other position on the staff of the American Nursing Home Association. (Charged by the author page 183).

3. *Summary*

On page 192, the author states that the organization she works for has "devoted itself to exposing the high profits and financial manipulations in the (nursing home) industry." This entire book is devoted to prove this conclusion. Again it is clear that by industry she means all operators in the U.S. Toward this end she provides a central core of data on Eugene Woods, Dr. Bergman, Max Strauss and Joseph Kosow. All of these names are familiar to me because they surfaced in our 1965 hearings. I agree with Elliot Richardson that much of what she has is "old material" (page 125) going back as far as 1959, 1960 and 1962. The author provides little that we did not have in 1965. Unfortunately many of the manipulations these men indulged in are not crimes as Attorney General Brooke wrote.

-6-

I certainly do not excuse these men for what they did. I deplore their action. But at the same time I deplore an effort in this book to tie in extraneous data much of it misused or false to create inferences or conclusions that every nursing home operator in the Nation is another Woods or Kosow.

If this book is published, nursing home operators will have perhaps the first legitimate usage of their "isolated instances" speech as predicted on page 30. I believe the book will unfairly increase the fear in the public mind associated with nursing homes since it asserts (incorrectly) that there have been no improvements in the quality of care since the early 1960's. Moreover, publication of this book could undo, to a marked degree, much of the work done by the Subcommittee on Long-Term Care over the past 10 years. This is particularly true because the book structures many straw men that are then knocked down while leaving real issues untouched.

I feel strongly that the book should not be published in its present form. *I in no way wish to be associated with it. I request that any and all references and attributions to the Subcommittee on Long-Term Care be deleted.* I would suggest strongly that you reconsider the use of General Accounting Office studies. I intend to turn over to them my copy of the galley's to the GAO for an examination of the misuse of their publications. Finally, if the book is published substantially unchanged, I shall denounce it with full vigor.

I have not arrived at these views hastily. I have consulted at least a dozen individuals whose expertise, advice and counsel I value in these matters. We are unanimous in the above views. *I emphasize that the above criticisms are but representative of the numerous errors and misstatements that permeate the book.* Counsel Halamandaris prepared a 14 page memorandum in reviewing the book at my request. I am sure that he would provide you with additional details should you so desire.

My closing statement to you is that Mrs. Mendelson and I are both critics of the industry and that as such we have the responsibility to be fair and honest. This book is neither.

With best wishes to you and Regina Ryan.

Sincerely,

Frank E. Moss

Chairman, Subcommittee

on Long-Term Care

Enclosure

cc: Honorable Edward Brooke, U.S. Senate

Comptroller General, Elmer Steers

The following is a letter from Senator Frank Moss to Thomas Bell, Executive Director of the American Nursing Home Association, June 26, 1974.

Dear Tom:

I am aware of the book, "Tender Loving Greed" by Mary Adelaide Mendelson that you referred to in your letter of June 21st. The manuscript was submitted to me and read in full by Val Halamandaris, who has worked with me on the Committee on Long-Term Care. We were aghast at some of the allegations of the book, and Val composed a really tough letter to the publisher. I'll enclose a copy of that letter so that you can see what we think of the book. I have not changed my opinion and I am shocked at the wide publicity that I have seen on this publication. Of course, a shocking or scandalous thing draws customers, so I suppose Mrs. Mendelson will profit from her efforts.

In the meantime, I have prepared a manuscript that I am now submitting to a publisher on the same general subject, but which I think is totally fair. I hope that it will be published and perhaps stand as something of a counter weight to the one by Mrs. Mendelson

Sincerely,

Ted Moss [signature]

Frank E. Moss

United States Senator

Finally, this is Val Halamandaris's letter to David Bain at Knopf, January 8, 1974, which included the fourteen page memo prepared for Moss.

Emphasis is in the original. The photocopy of the memo contains hand written annotations and corrections. Added words are indicted "["word" in pencil]" or emphasis "[emphasis in pencil]". I have ignored simple corrections that correct typographical errors, for example "her*f*". I do not actually know that these were made in pencil or pen, rather, saying "pencil" is a convenience.

Dear Mr. Bain:

Senator Moss requested that I make available to you the memorandum which I prepared for him after having read the draft of Mrs. Mendelson's proposed book. I am sending this memo along. I was somewhat reluctant to do so because of the rough nature of the writing. I employed several shorthand terms which I knew the Senator would understand.

I had hoped that you would call me directly for my views and that I could use these notes to construct a full reply. I will say simply that I heartily concur with Senator Moss's analysis. I do hope that you took the trouble to send the draft to Senators Charles Percy, Harrison Williams and Frank Church.

I enclose the memorandum you requested with my best wishes.

Sincerely

Val J. Halamandaris
Associate Counsel
Enclosure

[Memo Pg. 1]

Memo
To Senator
From: Val
Re; [sic] Mendleson's [sic] proposed book

That does it. I am going to write my own book if and when we ever get that damn report published. If a high class outfit like Knopf will publish this pile of garbage ["," in pencil] they will publish anything.

I agonized over this draft ["book" in pencil] for several days. I can see why you were so concerned. What makes it difficult for me is that she writes from the point of view of so many of my own prejudices. I feel that a great many nursing home operators are profiteering and there are some substantial abuses. I would be the last to say that *all* are bums. Her sweeping indictment of the whole industry will not wash.

My second big objection is in the casual way that she throws the Subcommittee name around. She asserts among other things that the GAO confirmed leads that she gave the Committee back in 1965. You know differently and so do I. They found a *few* examples of abuse not the state-wide everybody-is-doing-it kind of charge that she leveled. She has no business saying that she contributed in any substantial way to the Committee's April 1971 Chicago investigations. Moreover, she is all wet in asserting *for you* [emphasis in pencil] that you were dissatisfied with Brooke's investigation of Kosow leads. To

[Memo Pg. 2]

the best of my knowledge you never accused Brooke of playing patsy. I don't know anything about proposed contributions that Brooke is reputed to have received from nursing home interests. Do you know anything? Why not ask him outright. Myself, I am inclined to accept his statement as written to you in 1965 that there was no evidence to support a criminal indictment.

My third comment is that she is heading for the same trouble with this book that she ran into with her GEOMET Report. She represented the GEOMET report and her summary of it as proof, at long last, that the industry was profiteering. I am glad you excercised [sic] caution and had the GAO look at her material.

As you remember she took the GEOMET study which was a nice *hypothetical* [emphasis in pencil] that it was possible to make large profits while meeting existing standards *accompanied by variables and qualifications* [emphasis in pencil]---She forgot about the variables and the qualifications and in her summary of the report and press release made a flat statement that all nursing homes were making huge profits. She even forgot about ["it being a" in pencil] the ["the" crossed out in pencil] hypothetical.

As you recall the GAO gave us a report that made her, [sic] look like the damn fool she must be. I intervened asking the GAO not to be so harsh because I beleive [sic] in nice little old ladies. They soften ["ed" added in pencil] their criticism of her. I then sought to persude [sic] Mary that she could save face by stating the entire
[Memo Pg. 3]
report was only a hypothetical and that she would have done better if the industry had surrendered their own data on costs. Her acceptance of this position probably saved her from suit by GEOMET for what she did with their report (if not from the Nursing Home Association people) [parentheses in pencil]. You'll remember she sent h*er summary of the GEOMET rep*ort and all its assertions to every State Health Department and to about every reporter in town.

I assert that the book does the same thing, forgets about all the variables and qualifications each of which can change the result in an effort to make flat statements., [sic] I don't ["Think" in pencil] this procedure can be justified in an effort to sell books. The world simply isn't black and white.

Fourth, in the last part of her book she asserts that everywhere she turned no one listened. She recounts her appearance before the Grand Jury which came to nothing and she talks about inaction in the face of the GEOMET report. HER [caps in original] draft ignores much of legislation in reform of some of these alleged abuses. HR1, for example, has a provision making kickbacks illegal and punishing with a year in jail and $10,000 fine. I restate again that she circulated her summmary [sic] of the report not the report itself. What do you do when her facts just don't check out and when she overstates the case as she did with the GEOMET/ Federation Report and Press Release. Remember the stuff on the Marietta fire she gave us?

[Memo Pg. 4]

God save us from the reformers who see each and every proviors [sic] as a profiteer- they are just as bad as the members of the industry who assert that there is nothing wrong.

Five, it strikes me that the entire book is an effort to prove the profiteering thesis. She is convinced of a point of view and tries to prove it. Her evidence I think is scanty. Flat statements made again and again ending in conclusions mixed with a few dated examples of abuse. Our report differs in the sense that we gathered together the material and let the material dictate the direction of each chapter rather than starting from preconceived conclusions.

Sir, I tried to help these people last February. I spent four of five hours talking candidly with the guy that rewrote this thing. I encouraged them to go to the SEC and look up the profit data on all the 100 public nursing home chains so they could say something definitive about profits rather than inuendo [sic]. This was the only way they could get data to my knowledge. Nothing else is public. This they refused to do. As you know, I convinced myself that we needed this data and we spent most of the summer getting it. I provided them with the GAO plan of action on our 3 state ["profit study" in pencil] request. I told them about a sample of nursing homes in upstate New York that the GAO man had rounded up to varify [sic] return on investment figures.

[Memo Pg. 5]

I told them about the 450 percent return on investment figure to encourge [sic] them and tell them I felt that they were going in the right direction. I ["also" crossed out in pencil] told them this in confidence ["," in pencil] never dreaming that I would see it in print. This study was done informally as you know, it was never reduced to writing and could not be called a GAO product. The Comptroller General never signed off on any such report. All this I told them. Imagine my suprise [sic] to find the 450 percent figure used. We haven't used it in the report or publically [sic] anywhere else.

Another thing, they asked me if I knew about a Long on the payroll of the American Nursing Home Assn. I told them I had heard a rumor that Gillis Long was for a time on the payroll from the former secretary of ANHA. They also hired Bruce Thevenot whose brother works for Russell Long. I can't imagine their writing that Long has a nephew on the payroll of ANHA without checking it out further. The Congressman ["/" in pencil] Gillis is a distant relative if anything, to the best of my knowledge he isn't a consultant presently.

Moreover, I doubt that the American Nursing Home Association has much moxie with Russel [sic] Long. Their failure to get substanttive [sic] legislative goals last year with ["the" in pencil] Finance ["Committee" in pencil] proves the point. Long gave them a deaf ear in their request to have some of the tough language in HR1 deleted.

[Memo Pg. 6]

Seven, I am appalled by the charge she makes that *all* regulators are corrupt. A fur coat here and there, a Christmas turkey she asserts twists the heads of nursing home surveyors.

She asserts that HEW officials are not doing their jobs. That they demand impossible amounts of information. This reference relates to Mary's coming before various regulators with her charges. If the regulators did not put people in jail it was because they were lazy or on the take. The other alternative is more likely to me- that is that stuff she gave them did not check out.

The SEC didn't help her. The Grand Jury ["was fixed." in pencil] The State of Ohio., [sic] VA, the Senate, everyone is against her. Nobody listens. This being true her last resort is to write a book. What crap.

Her assertion that investigators demand impossible amounts of information is ridiculous. The fact that I was able to go to the SEC and get the profit data on the 100 public nursing home chains proves the point. She could have done that. It took me a long time to go throught [sic] it all because I was working and getting married etc [sic] but we did get concrete solid evidence. We offer no excuses. We offer facts not charges.

When our report is issued it will show other examples of the work of senior citizen volunteers working with us in nursing homes and the results of their work. An individual can improve the system. We listened to what they had

[Memo Pg. 7]

to tell us. Their data checked out.

Summary, This is the worst writing on nursing homes I have ever read. I think you should hit them and hit them hard. I had John Edie and our Counsel Dave Affeldt go over this stuff with me because of my great emotional involvement. They agree that the book is pathetic. I feel the book would do great damage to the credibility of nursing home critics. The nursing home industry will cut this thing to bits and pieces and rightly so. There is no room for error.

I will be more than glad to sit down with the publisher and show him chapter and verse. For your "edification" [quotation marks in pencil] I am including a page by page analysis. I have about 14 pages of written notes that are even harder to read. I trust you'll know what I am talking about from my criptic [sic] references.

I must say I don't enjoy the position of defending the nursing home industry. I honestly feel that this book is dishonest and overly sensational as well as ["crapy" in pencil]

I am at your disposal I will sit down and give you a more coherent draft if you'd like. Let me know you [sic] wishes.

[Memo Pg. 8]

Chapter 1.

From the very beginning this book asserts the nursing home industry is exploiting the poor aged and defrauding all of us. In short, it is a blanket indictment aimed at each and every operator in the nation. ["24/34 48, 129, 155" in pencil]

p. 17 Cadillac's [sic] are standard equipment in this business—assertion that all nursing home operators drive Cadillacs is repeated on pages, [sic] 34, 35, 106, 183. 186

Also on this page is a list of evils that Mary reportedly first learned from a Mr. Novak. "Everything he told me was confirmed many times over. . . ." Among the things he told her was that Las Vegas mone [sic], the mob, the mafia is involved in nursing homes. the [sic] author hints and suggest mafia envolement [sic] in nursing homes on pages 65, and 163 while admitting that no firm evidence exists on page 88. In truth no firm data exists; there are not even any good leads and it is wrong to give the impression that there are.

p. 18 The statement is made that there is no relationship between the dollars paid [sic] the quality of care. This same point is made throughout, see pages 29 and 36 [", 150" in pencil]. The statement is blatently [sic] false. This is recognized by the author on page 41 where paradoxically she asks for financial *incentives*.

p. 18 she also flatly asserts that providors [sic] (presumably *all* charge for non-delivered items) [sic] This is not true. It is presented without evidence. The data we have suggest that some are guilty but less than a majority.

p. 19 the authors give some idea of the methods they have employed such as hidden taperecorders [sic] as if nursing home operators are all criminals. I deplore this and all other inferences which are quickly drwn [sic] by the reader.

p. 20 reference to A [sic] chicago [sic] investigator and blank cards--should read an investigator of the Senate Subcommittee on Long-Term Care

21. Suggestion that all, or a majority or most nursing homes

work it so that all meals are compressed into one shift is blatantly false in our experience.

p. 22 Saying the food compared unfavorably with hospital food is a difficlut [sic] line to draw particularly for somebody like Mendelson who has had no hospital experience that I know of. In our experience the food in some hospitals is comparable.

[Memo Pg. 9]

p. 21 the generalization that it is rare for utinsils [sic] other than a spoon to be offered is ludicrous. That it is rare to see bread and butter is likewise ludicrous.

p. 22 that the average stay is 3 years in a nursing home is wrong - correct figures place it closer to two years than three.

p. 23 this 1967 list of ancillary charges is listed without telling of where it originated. No further, more current, or different list of such charges exist. They exist we are told because a 1972 publication by HEW warns the public to watch out for them. It misstates the nature of ancillary charges which are sometimes added on to the bill of private paying patients. It decries the administrators saying that Medicare will pay for 100 days care in our home. *In 1967 Medicare would pay for such care.* The rules were changing in 1969, so that almost no one qualifies for Medicare nursing home care now. Neither Medicare nor Medicaid patients pay ancillary charges ["only private paying." in pencil]

p. 26 an example Mr. Stua, what year was this? Conditions have chang[ed] drastically in last 10 years. No allowance has been made for these changes in the book.

p. ["29" in pencil] thievery and corruption in stinking nursing homes (again all ho[mes] under a blanket indictment) [Followed by something like, "The litigation for charges could be new_____ H.R. 1 Pub____ ____603." in pencil]

p. 29. Regulations make no difference she charges. Nursing homes are similar everywhere. This is grossly untrue. There are great differences between Connecticut homes for example and homes in Pennsylvania and Mississippi. Critical to the quality of care is both the reimbursement system and how it operates and the states regulatory procedures. Some states to [sic] a better job than others. No recognition of this fact is given.

p. 30 The industry will be right for once when they use the term isilated [sic] instances to describe this book. This is precisely what she has and has tried to build into a national indictment without further facts, without qualification—the whole effort is a hatchet job. Certainly not for Knopf publishers. Grove press, maybe.

p. 31 Other large scale exposes—beyond Nader? I know of none. The GAO reports hardly quality as large scale ["or as exposes." in pencil]

p. 31 She says for the first of three times that the GAO report in 1966 Confirmed [sic] her findings in the state of Ohio. I can only say baloney. They found a few examples of what she was talking about but you can read that GAO report and interpret it anyway that you want to.

[Memo Pg. 10]

p. 49 "An official testified he was offered a bribe of 100 a head" [sic] The implication is that he was a health officer in office and in charge during the hearings. Jack was temporarily in chage [sic] of the program to discharge mental patient [sic] into the Community.

Chapter Three

p. 65 invokes Subcommittee name should make it clear who is talking, (Frantz) [parentheses in pencil] or write in *former* Staff member.

This stuff on Woods is old as the hills, 1965 and before although she has done her best to keep it alive. The VA filed to follow up on the fine leads she provided. The Ohio Governor failed, only she kept up the battle. Is it not possible that the evidence to convict somebody (Woods) of a crime was just not there. Question: How many nursing homes did Woods have? Weren't most retirement hotels? Do you remember?

Chapter Four

Max Strauss. Interesting but more ancient history. Her projection from padding of a $7,000 claim by 23 percent applied nationally projecting a $800 million loss is extremely weak.

Two assertions are made: One-Medicare and Medicaid both pay claims submitted by operators; this is widespread [sic] Two-That operators convert social security checks belonging to patients to their. [sic] own use.

Little evidence is offered to support either in the book. Our evidence and the GAO audit done for us following up their California study in duplicate payments shows they are few and far between and most are recovered. Part of the reason is that Medicare is not paying off like it used to. Only 70,000 patients on any given day have their care paid for by Medicare.

There is little hard data on the misappropriation of social securit[y] checks or of the monthly cigarette money. What there is has not been invoked here. All we have is a bald conclusion.

From these isolated instances grows the generalization "these operators have their counterparts all over the nation". [sic] p.85

Chapter 5 Ownership

More ancient history on our friend Dr. Bergman 1965, 66 and 68 They really miss the point in this chapter. The [sic] blast HEW for not enforcing Moss amdenment [sic] requiring that those with 10 percent interest in nursing homes disclose such interest. States now comply. HEW has done its job. No mention of our amendment to HR1 last year to include all interests including mortgage [sic] interests [sic]

[Memo Pg. 11]

The loophole is still ["open" in pencil] for those with less than a 10 percent interest. They are off base when they say ownership is hidden so as to facilitate a sale and lease back arrangement. ["That" crossed out. "Moreover sales – leasing" penciled in] is perfectly legal tax device used openly by the best of companies.

1959, 61 data

Enter our friend Kosow. Remember him from 1965? They assert that money lenders today chrge [sic] nursing homes exhorbitant [sic] interests (40 percent). Who in their right mind would pay 40 percent today when you can get a bank laon [sic] for 10 or an FHA for 8. What about the effect of intervening truth in lending laws.? [sic] Can Kosow still operate in the old way today especially in New York? I doubt it.

They charge Brooke and Richardson wehn [sic] Mass Atty General failed to act on Kosow leads. I am inclined to beleive [sic] Brooke when he told the Committee that he did not have probative facts to support a criminal indictment. Richardson was right it is old material. I object to their stating *that the Subcommittee* thought the reason that Brooke might have backed off was campaign contribution from nursing home interests. If they want to charge that let them but don't put that in our mouth. The Subcommittee is 12 Senators last time I heard.

p. 118 Wells was grad student at Rutgers, his product is not that of Federal REserve [sic] Bank as represented here.

p. 127 A subcommittee staff member—say *former* staff member and identify.

Chapter 7

Page 129. Owners proclaim their profitability. Flat charge high profits, inflated costs. ["Book" penciled in] States flatly owners of chains usually own other companies, usually finance or construction. No facts just inference.

Less debt and more homes = more profit. Not true. More pretax profit maybe. Large debt equal expenses and deductions maybe more after-tax money. Naive analysis. P. 131.

138. Bergman-Kosow connection tenuous-[" " in pencil] involved in, associated with e [remainder of word missing] So little evidence that nursing home industry is in hands of a few. But this is common assertion. Damnit, [sic] it maybe true but prove it don't just charge it.

Chapter 8 Ancillary Services

Medicaid drugs $200 million one half padded. How absurd without proof. P.144

[Memo Pg. 12]

California study found kickbacks in vast majority of homes. ["(?)" in pencil] Small sample GAO the same thing. Another Minnesota study? What study? GAO reports do no say what they are reported to say.

Battle over brand names and generics is settled—author says there is no difference in quality. I'd like to know her credentials for making this judgment. 146

p. 146 RX instead of supply included in homes general rate— Says she has noticed homes give patients Darvon rather than aspirin because on [sic] is paid for by state. Wrong. both are paid if you can get a doctor to prescribe them.

p.147 DK Krause did not say that 25 percent of homes had drug problems. She said 25 t- [sic] 30 percent of homes had serious violations.

p. 147 they use a quote from Ellen Marx (unnamed) that is false and discredited in State hearing.

p. 145 They quote me incorrectly. I said 40 percent of drugs paid for by Medicaid were central nervous system drugs sedatives, tranquilzers [sic] and analgesics (aspirin) Sedatives about 4 percent, tranquilizers 19 percent and aspirin etc about 17 percent.

p.151 they give the impression that in most states doctors arerequired to view bodies of patients that have died before signing death certificates. This is false only about two states require it.

p. 151 They quote data 35 MDs collected $3 million from Medicaid and one got $131,000--This might be Medicaid but is it nursing homes? Again 11 dentists got 1 million. Is this nursing homes? I doubt it! The bigger problem is to get DRs to come to nursing homes not overutilization !!!

p. 155 Author aays [sic] Govt remains Inactive [sic]. What about HR1 past last year an specifically Section 242 banning kickbacks and setting up fines for misstatments [sic] and fraud of Medicare and Medicaid claims.

Chapter 9 Non Proftos [sic]

P. 163 "They are not significatly [sic] different from for profits given the genral [sic] level of dishonesty in the industry." [quotation marks in pencil] I say BS. Baumgarten is used as example of sale and lease back, Miller as

[Memo Pg. 13]

example of requiring family to subsidize Medicaid payments.

Baumgarten is involved in Troy Hills and Cranford Nursing Center. Both ["home are an" in pencil] architectural achievements in nursing home field.

They are wrong about Barmgarten [sic] being in Florida. He is in Denver. He did not have the influence on govenment [sic] policy they repute to him.

There is nothing illegal about the sale and lease back arrangement that either he or Miller used. The Miller subsidization of Medicaid which was alleged but not proved is illegal.

Ten

"Government is corrupt or indolent." [quotation marks in pencil] There is no pressure except from the industry. How false. What about Senir [sic] Citizen groups? ["AFL-CIO" in pencil] Investigators demand impossible amounts of data, her study and the GAO were a rout; as evidenced by the fact that 81 homes were closed asserted jury forman [sic]—(closed voluntarily perhaps.) Grand jury dismissed her investigation. State legislature wasn't impressed. Nursing homes got 40 percent increase as a result of lobbying. What about increase in costs. ["_____ enough for anybody." in pencil, first word unclear]

p. 180 HEW undertaking study of costs not profits.

p. 183 IRS some manuevers [sic] legal; audits drs withmore [sic] than $25,000; ["they" in pencil] audit Slader, Cohen, and selected nhs.

183 Nephew of Russel [sic] Long maybe distant relative not nephew

184 Everything tied up to indolence of gvt employees, po-

litical power of industry. What happens when the data you provide just doesn't work out.

188 "Training isn't important" [quotation marks in pencil] ["contrary to" in pencil] p.19 "you needed training to learn what to look for." [quotation marks in pencil] 2 more ombudsman programs now ["_____ created?" in pencil, first word unclear]

191 Great many ["people" in pencil] don't belong in nhs. Many do who are outside, [sic]

191 Political rights of patients meaningless—Like hell right to sue ["most critical" in pencil]

192 facts like hell—inuendos [sic]

194 Gvt remained silent ["if we had acted we would have had to _____ Mendelson for what she did to the Geomet report." in pencil, one word unclear]

The following photocopies of the preceding letters are also available, full-size, at:
http://www.12on14.com/site-images/moss-letters.pdf

United States Senate
SPECIAL COMMITTEE ON AGING
Washington, D.C. 20510

DEC 5 1973

Mr. David Bain
Assistant to Mrs. Regina Ryan
Editor
Alfred A. Knopf Publishers
201 East 50th Street
New York, New York 10022

Dear Mr. Bain:

Thank you and Mrs. Ryan for an opportunity to comment on the proposed book, Tender Loving Greed, by Mary Adelaide Mendelson. I appreciate the kind words about me and the work of my Subcommittee on Long-Term Care. I sincerely wish that I could tell you that this manuscript is accurate, constructive and an intelligent contribution to the battle we have been waging to improve life for the one million Americans who suffer the compound burdens of illness and advanced age.

In fact, the book is far from accurate. There are errors in the book too numerous to mention. Facts are few and far between. Inferences and generalizations abound. It gives currency to rumors that are sometimes outright lies. Piling inference on top of inference it reaches conclusions that are as absurd as to be humorous. In short, it lacks integrity and for this reason it is a very distructive writing. I don't know when I have been more disappointed and distressed. Here are a few examples of what I mean:

1. Inaccurate Generalizations

From the very beginning the book asserts the nursing home industry is exploiting the patient and defrauding all of us. There is no room left for doubt that the author's criticism is leveled at each and every operator in the U.S. These charges are made on page 24, 34, 29, 48, 129, 155. On page 30 the author states, "It disturbs me that I seem to be indicting all nursing homes with one sweep of the brush." She goes on to say that she has been in 200 homes and only seen one good one. On page 157, she notes that non-profit homes are "not significantly different from profit homes." The book, in short, is a blanket indictment of an entire industry.

Comment: This is a blatantly false premise that runs through the entire book. All nursing home operators are not dishonest any more than all politicians are on the take. Applying another analogy, it is like saying that all Italians are members of the Mafia. More such hasty generalizations follow.

Mr. David Bain   -2-

• It is alleged (as noted above) that all operators are making "incredible profits" (p.48,34,24,129,155), that there is "thievery and corruption in our stinking nursing homes".

Comment: Our studies show that it is almost impossible to generalize about nursing home profits. Some operators are making large profits and some are going broke. Goals and expectations differ. Operators set different goals, some seek to maximize equity, some seek to minimize equity. Some seek high profits before taxes, others seek after tax profits. Some actively seek tax losses with which to offset taxable gains in other business. Just as these expectations differ, their ability to reach them expectations differ. The results of our studies will be made public soon. The Department of HEW is undertaking a separate study (contrary to what was said on p.160) of nursing home profits and costs. The results of this study show that there is not much difference in cost across the nation between the average for a skilled nursing home and an intermediate care facility (less than a dollar per day per on the average). This is contrary to the author's statement (top of page 43) that intermediate care facilities "cost...a little more than half...that of a skilled nursing home."

• P.17, "Cadillacs are standard equipment for this business" -- asserting that all nursing home operators drive Cadillacs as a result of high profits. Assertion repeated p.34,35,106,143,186.

Comment: This is a ridiculous and untrue conclusion.

• Paraphrasing: "The Mafia is involved in nursing homes," p.17,65,163.

Comment: In 10 years of investigation we have never uncovered a scintilla of hard evidence to support such a statement. This the author admits on page 88, but the inferences in other sections of the book are allowed to stand.

The statement was made on page 18, that there is no relationship between the dollars paid and the quality of care. See also pages 29,36,155.

Comment: This is false. The reimbursement system and the amount of money States pay for welfare patients is the most important factor in the quality of care according to a study by Dr. Nancy Anderson, University of Minnesota, cited by the authors in a different context on page 159.

• On page 29 the author states that "regulations make no difference" and that nursing homes are similar everywhere and "similarly bad" in every State of the Union.

Comment: The conclusion is patently ridiculous. There are great differences in the quality of care offered in various States in the Union. Regulations and the type of State enforcement policies differ. Connecticut requires one registered nurse for every 30 patients on the day shift, one for every 45 on the afternoon units and one for every 60 on the night shift. The Federal standard is only one RN on the 7 a.m. to 3 p.m. shift and the minimum of a LPN in charge on the other

Mr. David Bain   -3-

two shifts. Many States do not even meet these Federal minimums. The quality of care in Mississippi, Pennsylvania and Massachusetts is far different from Connecticut.

• On page 18 another recurrent theme occurs, that all providers charge for non-delivered services. The assertion is repeated in many places throughout Chapter 8.

Comment: All providers (suppliers would be a better word) do not seek to defraud the government. Contrary to the assertion in Chapter 8 that cause involving "ancillary charges" are the most well documented examples of fraud and corruption, I have seen little evidence of abuse concerning morticians, linen suppliers, or ambulance drivers. I have seen precious little in physicians. What evidence there is relates to drug kickbacks. Even where the evidence is contradictory. The good evidence that is available is not cited in the book. There is no new evidence on the activities of any other suppliers. On page 151, there is a reference to the fact that 35 doctors collected 53 million from Medicaid and that eleven dentists collected $1 million. The reference is oblique, implying that this happened in nursing homes. My instincts tell me that the citation refers to the Medicaid program in general of which nursing homes are a small part.

The few references to physicians' "gang visits" are accurate but we feel this is not a significant problem in view of the IRS corrective action. IRS action was apparently missed by the author who blasts them for non-action on page 143. IRS automatically audits the returns of physicians with incomes over $25,000 who have substantial claims coming from Medicare and Medicaid. Medicare and Medicaid send duplicate vouchers with the physician number to IRS. We have found that the bigger problem is to get doctors to go to nursing homes rather than in doctors providing care that isn't needed.

• The author states on page 157, that there is very little difference between non-profit and for profit homes, implying that both are bad.

Comment: It is certainly true that some homes use non-profit status as a guise. It is also true that most do not. In my experience, the best homes in the U.S. are church owned, related and operated and therefore non-profit. I am willing to contend that there are no significant differences between for-profit and non-profit homes. There are some significant studies which show more staff in non-profit homes, higher salaries for employees and lower turnover rates for aides and employees. Against this, the author offers one Minnesota study and two examples. Chapter 9 is extremely weak.

2. A few Obvious Errors

A. The author's use of General Accounting Office audits is extremely casual. A few examples:

Page 32 "GAO turned up swindles in six other States," among them Oklahoma, Michigan, and New York. This is an obvious reference to the May 26, 1971 audit

Mr. David Bain   -4-

of these three States. The audit measures whether fire safety, physicians and nursing standards were being met and points out a lack of a uniform definition of skilled nursing care in the 50 States.

On page 42 the author uses this same report to argue that many people are in nursing homes who don't belong there. "GAO concluded...that 90 percent of the patients in Michigan did not need nursing care."

Comment: GAO stated that when one set of criteria was applied 42 percent of the patients in Michigan did not need skilled nursing care. When another set of criteria were applied 79 percent did not need skilled nursing care. It did not say that they did not need nursing home care, just that there was no uniform definition and that some people needed a different level of nursing home care.

• Page 32, the author asserts that GAO is doing a study of profits in Oregon and Florida.

Comment: GAO and the Committee staff completed a study of Tennessee, Massachusetts, and Colorado for our forthcoming report. There is no study of Oregon and Florida according to my information.

• Page 36, there is an assertion that GAO has undertaken a study showing nursing homes with a 450 percent return on investment in five years.

Comment: There is no such study according to my information.

B. The Invocation of the Subcommittee Name

The name of the Subcommittee on Long-Term Care is used on several occasions. Attributions are made to the Subcommittee and its staff which should not be made. On page 105,124,125, and 128, it is asserted that the Subcommittee pressured intervention with respect to Mr. Krome or the then Attorney General of Massachusetts, Edward Brooke. The book charges that the Attorney General did not conduct a vigorous investigation. This charge is attributed to me rather than the author, e.g. "The Subcommittee thought that the answer might lie in campaign contributions (to the Brooke-for-Senator campaign)."

Comment: The Subcommittee is made up of myself and 16 other members of the Senate (1941). I have never leveled such a charge and to the best of my recollection neither did any other member of the Committee. I doubt any member of the staff made any such statement. Moreover, the staff members are without authority to make such a charge. To this day I suspect Senator Brooke's statement to me that he was "not in possession of sufficient probative facts to state that these irregular and questionable actions were of a criminal nature."

C. Other Errors

• On page 147 the book uses a quote from an unnamed person, (Ellen Marx)

Mr. David Bain   -5-

who appeared at our Minnesota hearings. This witness was greatly discredited in follow-up hearings held by the State.

Mrs. Daphne Krause did not testify that 25 percent of nursing homes have drug problems. She said about 25-30 percent of the homes in Minnesota had serious abuses some of which were drug problems.

On page 145 the author misquotes Associate Counsel Val J. Halamandaris of the Senate Special Committee on Aging. He stated that 40 percent of nursing home drugs were classified as central nervous system drugs. The author's language suggested Committee Counsel said that 40 percent of drugs were either tranquilizers or sedatives. This is not true. To be exact 19 percent are tranquilizers, about 10 percent are sedatives and another 10 percent are analgesics, including drugs like Darvon and aspirin.

This brings up another error, page 146 which charges nursing homes supply a prescription drug (Darvon) instead of an aspirin because the latter should be furnished as part of the homes general supplies. This is untrue. Both drugs are paid for by Medicaid if prescribed by a doctor (even in the State of Ohio) according to the GAO study for the Committee which Mr. Halamandaris cites.

Pages 159 and 170, Harold Baumgarten is charged with great influence on government nursing home policy. In reality, he had little. Some of the little influence he had might have even been counterproductive. For example, his Committee recommended in strong language that Nursing Home Licensure Boards set up by the States should not be dominated by the nursing home industry. Moreover, I am informed that he is in Denver and not Florida.

With respect to Dr. Miller in the same chapter, I am informed that the State of New York did have problems with the quality of care in the early days but that care is adequate to good at the present time. I have seen no proof that he subsidized Medicaid in violation of the law. I suggest the possibility of a libel suit here.

Senator Russell Long assures me that he has no nephew serving as counsel or in any other position on the staff of the American Nursing Home Association. (Charged by the author page 183).

3. Summary

On page 192, the author states that the organization she works for has "devoted itself to exposing the high profits and financial manipulations in the (nursing home) industry." This entire book is devoted to prove this conclusion. Again it is clear that by industry she means all operators in the U.S. Toward this end she provides a central core of data on Eugene Woods, Dr. Bergman, Max Strauss and Joseph Knowe. All of these names are familiar to me because they surfaced in our 1965 hearings. I agree with Elliot Richardson that much of what she has in "old material" (page 125) going back as far as 1959,1960 and 1962. The author provides little that we did not have in 1965. Unfortunately many of the manipulations these men indulged in are not crimes as Attorney General Brooke wrote.

Mr. David Bain   -6-

I certainly do not excuse these men for what they did. I deplore their action. But at the same time I deplore an effort in this book to tie in extraneous data much of it misused or false to create inferences or conclusions that every nursing home operator in the Nation is another Woods or Knowe.

If this book is published, nursing home operators will have perhaps the first legitimate usage of their "isolated instances" speech as predicted on page 30. I believe the book will unfairly increase the fear in the public mind associated with nursing homes since it asserts (incorrectly) that there have been no improvements in the quality of care since the early 1960's. Moreover, publication of this book could undo, to a marked degree, much of the work done by the Subcommittee on Long-Term Care over the past 10 years. This is particularly true because the book structures many straw men that are then knocked down while leaving real issues untouched.

I feel strongly that the book should not be published in its present form. I in no way wish to be associated with it. I request that any and all references and attributions to the Subcommittee on Long-Term Care be deleted. I would suggest strongly that you reconsider the use of General Accounting Office studies. I intend to turn over to them my copy of the galley's to the GAO for an examination of the misuse of their publications. Finally, if the book is published substantially unchanged, I shall denounce it with full vigor.

I have not arrived at these views hastily. I have consulted at least a dozen individuals whose expertise, advice and counsel I value in these matters. We are unanimous in the above views. I emphasize that the above criticisms are but representative of the numerous errors and misstatements that permeate the book. Counsel Halamandaris prepared a 14 page memorandum in reviewing the book at my request. I am sure that he would provide you with additional details should you so desire.

My closing statement to you is that Mrs. Mendelson and I are both critics of the industry and that as such we have the responsibility to be fair and honest. This book is neither.

With best wishes to you and Regina Ryan.

Sincerely,

Frank E. Moss
Chairman, Subcommittee
on Long-Term Care

Enclosure

cc: Honorable Edward Brooke, U.S. Senate
    Comptroller General, Elmer Staats

FRANK E. MOSS
UTAH

United States Senate
WASHINGTON, D.C. 20510

June 24, 1974

Thomas G. Bell
Executive Vice-President
American Nursing Home Assn.
1200-15th Street, N. W.
Washington, D. C. 20005

Dear Tom:

I am aware of the book, "Tender Loving Greed", by Mary Adelaide Mendelson that you referred to in your letter of June 21st. The manuscript was submitted to me and read in full by Val Halamandaris, who has worked with me on the Committee on Long-Term Care. We were aghast at some of the allegations of the book, and Val composed a really rough letter to the publisher. I'll enclose a copy of that letter so that you can see what we think of the book. I have not changed my opinion and I am shocked at the wide publicity that I have seen on this publication. Of course, a shocking or scandalous thing draws customers, so I suppose Mrs. Mendelson will profit from her efforts.

In the meantime, I have prepared a manuscript that I am now submitting to a publisher on the same general subject, but which I think is totally fair. I hope that it will be published and perhaps stand as something of a counterweight to the one by Mrs. Mendelson.

Sincerely,

Frank E. Moss
United States Senator

FEM:lj

United States Senate

SPECIAL COMMITTEE ON AGING
WASHINGTON, D.C. 20510

January 8, 1976

Mr. David Bain
Alfred A. Knopf Incorporated
201 East 50th Street
New York, New York 10022

Dear Mr. Bain:

Senator Moss requested that I make available to you the nomination which I prepare for him after having read the draft of Mrs. Mendieson's proposed book. I am sending this memo along. I was somewhat reluctant to do so because of the rough nature of the writing. I explained several shorthand terms which I knew the Senator would understand.

I had hoped that you would call me directly for my views and that I could use these notes to construct a full reply. I will say simply that I heartily concur with Senator Moss's analysis. I do hope that you took the trouble to send the draft to Senators Charles Percy, Harrison Williams and Frank Church.

I enclose the memorandum you requested with my best wishes.

Val J. Halamandaris
Associate Counsel

Enclosure

Memo

To: Senator
From: Val
Re: Mendieson's proposed book

That does it. I am going to write my own book if and when we ever get that damn report published. If a high class outfit like Knopf will publish this pile of garbage, they will publish anything.

I agonized over this draft for several days. I can see why you were so concerned. What makes it difficult for me is that she writes from the point of view of so many of my own prejudices. I feel that a great many nursing home operators are profiteering and there are some substantial abuses. I would be the last to say that *all* are bums. Her sweeping indictment of the whole industry will not wash.

My second big objection is in the casual way that she throws the Subcommittee name around. She asserts among other things that the GAO confirmed leads that she gave the Committee back in 1965. You know differently and so do I. They found a *few* examples of abuse not the state-wide everybody-is-doing-it kind of charge that she leveled. She has nb business saying that she contributed in any substantial way to the Committee's April 1971 Chicago investigations. Moreover, she is all wet in asserting for you that you were dissatisfied with Brooks's investigation of Kosow leads. To

the best of my knowledge you never accused Brooke of playing patsy. I don't know anything about proposed contributions that Brooke is reputed to have received from nursing home interests. Do you know anything? Why not ask him outright. Myself, I am inclined to accept his statement as written to you in 1965 that there was no evidence to support a criminal indictment.

My third comment is that she is heading for the same trouble with this book that she ran into with her GAO report. She represented the GAO report and her summary of it as proof, at long last, that the industry was profiteering. I am glad you exercised caution and had the GAO look at her material.

As you remember she took the GAO study which was a nice hypothetical that it was possible to make large profits while meeting existing standards accompanied by variables and qualifications---She forgot about the variables and the qualifications and in her summary of the report and press release made a flat statement that all nursing homes were making huge profits. She even forgot about the hypothetical.

As you recall the GAO gave us a report that made her look like the damn fool she must be. I intervened asking the GAO not to be so harsh because I believe in nice little old ladies. They softened their criticism of her. I then sought to persuade Mary that she could save face by stating the entire

report was only a hypothetical and that she would have done better if the industry had surrendered their own data on costs. Her acceptance of this position probably saved her from suit by GEOGET for what she did with their report if not from the Nursing Home Association people. You'll remember she sent her summary of the GEOGET report and all its assertions to every state Health Department and to about every reporter in town.

I assert that the book does the same thing, forgets about all the variables and qualifications each of which can change the result in an effort to make flat statements. I don't think this procedure can be justified in an effort to sell books. The world simply isn't black and white.

Fourth, in the last part of her book she asserts that everybody who turned no one listened. She recounts her appearance before the Grand Jury which came to nothing and she talks about inaction in the face of the GEOGET report. HEW draft ignores much of legislation in reform of some of these alleged abuses. HR1, for example, has a provision making kickbacks illegal and punishing with a year in jail and $10,000 fine. I restate again that she circulated her summary of the GEOGET report not the report itself. What do you do when her facts just don't check out and when she overstates the case as she did with the GEOGET/Federation Report and Press Release. Remember the stuff on the Marietta fire she gave us?

God save us from the reformers who see each and every provisor as a profiteer— they are just as bad as the members of the industry who assert that there is nothing wrong.

Five, it strikes me that the entire book is an effort to prove the profiteering thesis. She is convinced of a point of view and tries to prove it. Her evidence I think is scanty. Flat statements made again and again ending in conclusions mixed with a few dated examples of abuse. Our report differs in the sense that we gathered together the material and let the material dictate the direction of each chapter rather than starting from preconceived conclusions.

Six, I tried to help these people last February. I spent four of five hours talking candidly with the guy that re-wrote this thing. I encouraged them to go to the SEC and look up the profit data on all the 100 public nursing home chains so they could say something definitive about profits rather than innuendo. This was the only way they could get data to my knowledge. Nothing else is public. This they refused to do. As you know, I convinced myself that we needed this data and we spent most of the summer getting it. I provided them with the GAO plan of action on our 3 state request. I told them about a sample of nursing homes in upstate New York that the GAO men had rounded up to verify return on investment figures.

I told them about the 450 percent return on investment figure to encourage them and tell them I felt that they were going in the right direction. I also told them this in confidence, never dreaming that I would see it in print. This study was done informally as you know, it was never reduced to writing and could not be called a GAO product. The Comptroller General never signed off on any such report. All this I told them. Imagine my surprise to find the 450 percent figure used. We haven't used it in the report or publicly anywhere else.

Another thing, they asked me if I knew about a Long on the payroll of the American Nursing Home Assn. I told them I had heard a rumor that Gillis Long was for a time on the payroll of ANHA. They also hired Bruce Thevenot whose brother works for Russel Long. I can't imagine their writing that Long has a nephew on the payroll of ANHA without checking it out further. The Congressman/Gillis is a distant relative if anything, to the best of my knowledge he isn't a consultant presently.

Moreover, I doubt that the American Nursing Home Association has much moxie with Russel Long. The/it failure to get substantitive legislative goals last year with Finance proves the point. Long gave them a deaf ear in their request to have some of the tough language in H.1 deleted.

Seven, I am appalled by the charge she makes that all regulators are corrupt. A fur coat here and there, a Christmas turkey she asserts twists the heads of nursing home surveyors.

She asserts that HEW officials are not doing their jobs. That they demand impossible amounts of information. This reference relates to Mary's coming before various regulators with her few facts and bountiful charges. If the regulators did not act weren't put in jail it was because they were lazy or on the take. The other alternative is more likely to me: that is that the stuff she gave them did not check out.

The FBI didn't help her. The Grand Jury, the State of Ohio, VA, the Senate everyone is against her. Nobody listens. This being true her last resort is to write a book. What crap.

Her assertion that investigators demand impossible amounts of information is ridiculous. The fact that I was able to go to the SEC and get the profit data on the 100 public nursing home chains proves the point. She could have done that. It took me a long time to go through it all 'cause I was working and getting married etc but we did get concrete solid evidence. We offer no excuses. We offer facts not charges.

When our report is issued it will show other examples of the work of senior citizen volunteers working with us in nursing homes and the results of their work. An individual can improve the system. We listened to what they had

to tell us. Their data checks out.

Summary. This is the worst writing on nursing homes I have ever read. I think you should hit them and hit them hard. I had John Edie and our General Dave Affeldt go over this stuff with me because of my great emotional involvement. They agree that the book is pathetic. I feel the book would do great damage to the credibility of nursing home critics. The nursing home industry will eat this thing to bits and rightly so. There is no room for error.

I will be more than glad to sit down with the publisher and show I'm chapter and verse. For your edification as including a page by page analysis. I have about 14 pages of written notes that are even harder to read than my cryptic references.

I must say I don't enjoy the position of defending the nursing home industry. I honestly feel that this book is dishonest and overly sensationalistic as well as inaccurate.

I am at your disposal. I will sit down and give you a more coherent draft if you'd like. Let me know you wishes.

Chapter 1

From the very beginning this book asserts the nursing home industry is exploiting the poor aged and defrauding all of us. In short, it is a blanket indictment aimed at each and every operator in the nation.

p. 17 Cadillac's the standard equipment in this business--assertion that all nursing home operators drive cadillacs is repeated on pages, 34, 35, 106, 183, 184

Also on this page is a type of calls that Mary reportedly first learned from a Mr. Sowak. "Everything he told me was confirmed many times over...." Among the things he told her was that Las Vegas money, the mob, the mafia is involved in nursing homes. The enting hints and suggest mafia envolvement in nursing homes on pages 85, and 184 while admitting that no firm evidence exists on page 28. In truth no firm data exists, there are not even any good leads and it is wrong to give the impression that there are.

p. 18 The statement is made that there is no relationship between the dollars paid the quality of care. This same point is made ih roughout, see pages 29 and 76. The statement is blatantly false. This is recognized by the author on page 41 where paradoxically she asks for financial *incentives.*

p. 18 she also asks flatly asserts that providers (presumably all charge for non-delivered items) This is not true. It is presented without evidence. The data we have suggest that some are guilty but less than a majority.

p. 19 the authors give some idea of the methods they have employed such as hidden tonerecorders as if nursing home operators are all criminals. I despise this and all other inferences which are quickly drwn by the reader.

p. 20 reference to a chicago investigator and blank cards--should read an investigator of the Senate Subcommittee on Long-Term Care

21. Suggestion that all, or a majority or 80xxxxxxx most nursing homes work it so that all meals are compressed into one shift is blatantly false in our experience.

p.22 Saying the food compared unfavorably with hospital food is a difficult line to draw particularly for somebody like Mendelson who has had no hospital experience that I know of. In our experience the food in some hospitals is comparable.

p. 21 the generalization that it is rare for utensils other than a spoon to be offered is ludicrous. That it is rare to see bread and butter is likewise ludicrous.

p. 22 that the average stay is 3 years in a nursing home is wrong - correct figures place it closer to two years than three. 1967

p. 23 this lfist of ancillary charges is listed without telling of when it originated. To further, no current, or different list of such charges exist. They exist are sold because a 1972 publication by HEW says the public to watch out for them. It associates the extra and ancillary charge with are sometimes added on to the bill of private paying patients. It decries the administration saying that instead it will pay for 100 days care in our home... a 1977 Medicare would not for such care. The rules were changed so that no one qualifies for Medicare nursing home care now. Dmph Medicare nor Medicaid patients pay ancillary charges any more...

p. 26 an example is, that, which over are third conditions have changed dramatically over last 10 years. No allowance has been made for these changes in the book.

p. thievery and corruption in existing nursing homes (again all ho under a blanket indictment)...

p. 29, Regulations make no difference in charges. Nursing homes are similar everywhere. This is provable untrue. There are great differences between Connecticut homes for example and homes in Pennsylvania and Mississippi. Critical to the quality of care is both the reimbursement system and how it operates and the state regulatory procecesures. Some states to a better job than others. No recognition of this fact is given.

p. 30 The industry will be right for over when they use the term isilated 'nstances to describe this book. This is precisely what she has and has tried to build into a national indictment without further facts, without qualifications-- the whole effort is a hatchet job. Certainly not for Knopf publishers . Grove press, maybe.

p. 31 Other large scale crimmes --beyond Nader? I know of none. The GAO reports hardly qualify as large scale...

p. 31. She says for the first of three times the the Ax GAO report in 1966 confirmed her findings in the state of Ohio. I can only say between. They found a few examples of what she was talking about but you can can read that GAO report and interpret it anyway that you want to.

p, 49"An official testified he was offered a bribeof 100 a head" The implication is that he was a health officer in office and in charge du ing the huor nge. Shexxxxx Jack was temporarily in chage of the program to discharge mental patient into the Community. Chapter Three

p. 65 invokes Subcommittee name xxx should make it clear who is talking, (Frontv) or write in former staff member

This stuff on Woods is old as the hills, 1965 and before although she has done her best to keep it alive. The VA failed to follow up on the five leads she provided. The Ohio Governor failed, only she kept up the battle. Is it not possible that the evidence to convict somebody (Woods) of a crime was just not there. Question: How many nursing homes did Woods have? Weren't most retirement hotels? Do you remember?

Chapter Four

Max Strauss. Interesting but more ancient history. Her projection from the swndling of a $3,000 claim by 23 percent applied nationally projecting a $800 million loss is extremely weak.

Two assertions are made: One-Medicare and Medicaid both pay claims submitted by operators--is is ludicrous? Two-That operators convert social security checks belonging to patients to their own use.

Little evidence is offered to support either in the book. Our evidence and theGAO audit done for us following up on their California study in duplicate payments shows they are Few and far between and most are recovered. In fact of the reason is that Medicare is not paying all like it used to. Only 70,000 patients on any given day have their care paid for by Medicare.

There is little hard data on the misappropriation of social security checks or of the monthly cigarette money. What there is has not been invoked here. All we have is a kmxx bald conclusion.

From these isolated instances grows the xxxxxxxxx generalization "these operators have their counterparts all over the nation". p.85

Chapter 5 Ownership

More ancient history on our friend Dr. Bergman 1965, 66 and 68 They really miss the point in this chapter. The issue HEW for not enforing Moss amdmt bf requiring that those with 10 percent interest in nursing homes disclose such interest. States have comply. HEW has done its job. No mention of our amendment to HRl last year to include all interests including mortgage interests

The loophole is still, for those with less than a 10 percent interest. They are off base when they say ownership is hidden so as to facilitate a sale and lease back arrangement. That is perfectly legal tax device used openly by the best of companies. 1959 AI data

Enter our friend Kasow, November 15 1965? They assert that money lenders today chrge more on homes exhorbitant interest (all percent). Who in their right mind would pay 40 percent today when you can get a bank loan for 10 or so 75% for 8. What about the effect of intervening truth in lending laws? Can Kasow still operate in the old way today especially in New York? I doubt it.

They charge Smoke and Richardson were Mass Atty General failed to act on these leads. I am inclined to belive Brooke when he said the Connic.. riot he did not have xxxxx probtive facts to mount a criminal indictment, I disagree ith right 6t to old materials, a object to their stating that the Subcommittee thought the reason that Smoke eight have looked off was company corruption from nursing home interests. If they want to charge their let them but don't put that in oebehalf. The Subcommitt. is 12 Scnators last time I heard.

p.118' Needs was real student at Harvard, hi, product is not that of federal Rtserve B nk as questioned here.

p.127 A subcommittee staff member--say former staff member and identify.

Chapter 7. *Rech*

Page179, Owens proclaim their profitability. Flat charge high profits, inflated costs. State flatly owners of chains usualy own other companies, usually finance or construction. No facts just inference.

Less debt and more homes = more profit. Not true. More pretax profit maybe. Large debt equal expenses and deductions maybe more after-tax money. Save analysis. p. 131.

138. Bergman-Kasow condition remains-involved in, associated with e So little evidence that nursing home industry is in hands of a few. But this is common assertion. Doesn't.it may be true but p ove it don't just charge it.

Chapter 8 Ancillary Services

Medicaid drugs $700 million or half padded. How absurd without proof. p. 144

California study found kickbacks in vast majority of homes.(?)
Small sample GAO found the same thing. Another Minnesota
study? What study? GAO reports do not say what they are
reported to say.

Battle over brand names and generics is settled--author says
there is no difference in quality. I'd like to know her
creden ials for making this judgment. 146

p. 146 RX instead of supply included in house gneral rate--
Says she has noticed homes give patients Darvon rather than
aspiring because on is paid for by state. Wrong. both are paid
if you can get a doctor to prescribe them.

p. 147 DRAwouse did not say they 25 percent of homes had drug
problems. She said 25 t- 30 percent of homes had serious
violation

p. 147 they use a quote from Ellen Mara (unnamed) that is false
and discredited in Stae hearings.

145 They quote us incorrectly. I dama said 40 percent of
drugs paid for by Medicaid were central nervous system drugs
sedatives, tranquilizers and analgesics (aralgins). Sedatives about
4 percent, tranquilizers 19 percent and aspirin etc about 17
percent.

p. 151 they give the impression that in most states doctors are
required to view bodies of patients that have d ed before
signing dea h certificates. This is false only about two states
require it.

p. 151 They quote data 35 was collected 63 million from
Medicaid and augget $131,000-- This might be Medi aid but is
it nursing homes. Again 11 dentists got 1 million. Is this nursing
homes I doubt it! The bigger problem is to get DRs to come to
nursing homes not overutilization."

p.155 Author says Govt remains inact ve. What about HRI cost
last year on specifically Decimon 247 booming kickbacks and
setting up fines for misstatments and fraud of Medicare and Medicaid
claims.

Chapter 9 Non Profios

P. 163 "They are not significantly different from for profits
given the genral level of dishonesty in the industry." I say BS.
Baumgarten is used as example of sale and lease back, Miller as

example of requiring family to subsidize Medicaid payments.

Baumgarten is involved in Troy Hills and Cranford Nursing
Center. Both architectural achievements in nursing home field.

They are wrong about Baumgarten being in Florida. He is in Denver.
He did not have the influence on govenmen olicy they repute
to him.

There is no hing illegal about the sale and lease back
arrangement that either he or Miller used. The Miller subsidization
of Medicaid which was alleged but not proved is illegal.

Ten

Government is corrupt or indolear! There is no pressure except from
the industry. Not false. What about Gray Citizen groups, AFL-CIO
investigation, deided impossible in course of Aira, her study and
the GAO were wrong, as evidenced by the fact that 81 homes
were closed or taken over, only some expelled voluntarily perhaps.)
Grand Jury convened new investigation,State legislature wasn't
increased, nursing homes cut 63 percent increase as a result of
lobbying. What about increase inpests? In some enough for industry.

p. 180 HEW undertaking study of costs on profits

p. 183 HEW now empowers local; audits can withnold than 25,000; now
audit physician ,nurses, and related who.

183 Nephew of Daniel Langolistom relation not nephew
NYCS

184 Everything tied up to indolence of gov employees,political
power of industry. What happens when the data you provide
just doesn't work out.

185 Training isn't important p. 19 you needed training to learn what
to look for. I more subsidzed programs now for indicated.

191 Great many don;t belong in nhs. Many do who are outside.

191 Political rights of patients meaningless--Like hell right to sue
197 facts like hell --ismended most evident
198 Govt remained silent --if we had acted only
would have had a clearcut mandelion for
what she did to the Bronx hyest.

15

TLG in 2009

In the course of preparing this book, I have heard from several people who confirmed much of what I have read over the last few years: despite the many advances in medicine and what by now must be hundreds of thousands of regulatory pages written and disseminated since *TLG* was first published, despite many newer buildings, despite three and a half decades—the plight of the elderly in nursing homes has changed little. There is still some good, a lot of indifferent, and too much bad care. One profound difference, a sad difference, is that in the 1970s there was a sense that long-term care could be changed, that investigations and books could make a difference. As Mary Ad said,

> Only an angry public aware of the nature of the nursing home
> industry could affect a change; that transforming public interest
> could only be accomplished by a popular book.

but, if the current debate over health care (ObamaCare) is indicative, virtually no one mentions long-term care or nursing homes—and there are no popular books.

There are inklings in *TLG* and *CoS* that suggest that health care, in all its facets, is inhabited by the sons and grandsons of the men who stalked *TLG*. When we ask, "Why is health care so expensive?" perhaps there lies at least one significant explana-

327

tion. Does torte reform, which I think is an important issue—certainly it effects honest doctors who try to practice their craft of providing medicine—explain everything? The major pharmaceuticals must make a profit—to satisfy their stockholders and to fund the almost unimaginable costs attendant to developing new and better drugs. Insurance companies must make enough money to cover both ordinary and catastrophic risks, while remaining profitable. I'm sure that irregularities and distorted business practices abound, but do they explain the high costs?

We think of organized crime as Don Vito Corleone doing business from his estate. But from 1993 to 2006, the real godfather of the Corleonesi—and some have said the head of the Mafia—Bernardo Provenzano lived, as he had since 1963, in hiding. He spent his time hiding in little farms and when he was caught, he was living no better than the pigs. We think of gambling, prostitution, numbers, drugs. We think of the machine gunning of enemies. All true, but we forget, for example, the siphoning off of millions of dollars from banks through redirecting the small fractions of pennies, the residue of applying small percentage fees to every transaction. Consider that eBay honestly makes its money from adding a nickle here and dime there to every listed item. The nickels and dimes adds up.

We think of the movie producer Jack Woltz, in *The God-father*, waking to find his horse's head in his bed—the offer he couldn't refuse. But it doesn't have to be spectacular. I grew up with our phone lines tapped and frequent bomb threats. But the Justice Department Organized Crime people said they were probably not things to worry about. More powerful were the subtle threats: A Marlboro cigarette butt stamped out on Mary Ad's office floor when she opened the office on a Monday; a bottle of vodka that had turned yellow (the coroner's office analyzed it as "the urine of a young male"). You can't complain to the police, they would laugh: but you knew.

I talked about the staff, and its power. I don't believe that they were connected to crime. But through a wide and complicated net, they are subtly co-opted.

I do not believe that organized crime explains everything, nor does surveyors, investigators, staff or Congressmen being co-opted. But if the perception of the health care debate is about insurance companies, doctors performing unnecessary operations or tests, and drug company shenanigans—it is a false debate.

TLG opens a door to the deeper, more insidious and pernicious problems. When you listen to the experts talking about policies and regulatory difficulties, ask why they aren't talking about ownership, surveys, enforcement, reimbursement. Ask why fraud is serious, yet they talk about millions or billions, but not losses approaching a trillion dollars. Ask why the problems sound so *clean.*

Mary Ad felt that reimbursement for the honest health care provider is too low. For the crooks it's enough, and of course they would welcome more.

A final word on fraud. Fraud is "any act, expression, omission, or concealment calculated to deceive another to his or her disadvantage: a misrepresentation or concealment with reference to some fact material to a transaction that is made with knowledge of its falsity or in reckless disregard of its truth or falsity and with the intent to deceive another and that is reasonably relied on by the other who is injured" (<http://research.lawyers.com/fraud.html>). Therefore: ownership; tax, mortgage and loan manipulations; organized crime; co-opted regulators, staff, and legislators; and profiteering doctors, owners, and related providers come under that heading—whether organized or individual. Malcolm Sparrow's, *License to Steal: Why Fraud Plagues America's Health Care System*, explores part of that, and it is a book to be read. He does not talk about the staff nor, in any depth, organized crime. But lumped into this rubric, fraud and abuse, we can the find honest, well-meaning efforts of a doctor, for example, who in a community such as mine where the average age is over seventy, might want to routinely give his patients a throat culture to test for streptococcal infection. A simple and relatively low cost test. But if he gets back too many negative results, Medicare could refuse payment or disapprove him as a Medicare provider because of fraud and abuse. Or, if a doctor doesn't get paid by Medicare for months, perhaps as long as a year and a half, what does he do?

When politicians talk about fraud, be aware that those words too often are a gossamer fabric.

Thus, in 1977, the U.S. Attorney General, Griffin Bell, promised a Justice Department crackdown on fraud in the health care industry. Toward that end, he was training some FBI agents in the special field of Medicaid and Medicare. This promise seemingly did not go very far, if the hearing held by the Senate subcommittee in 1980 to receive testimony from the FBI is any indication.

At the hearing, the FBI agents estimated that 90 percent of the providers of the services were in some way corrupt. Kickbacks and inflated costs were a fact of life, they said. Some of the Senators placed the blame on HHS. Senator Dole produced a memo that revealed a negative approach by the Secretary Patricia Harris. She told her staff not to use the word *fraud* anymore and instead to label it "management inefficiency." Senator Packwood concluded that the department did not care about fraud or corruption: "Their job is to shovel out as much money as they can." If there is some fraud and corruption, it is just part of normal business, said the Senator. [CoS]

Regarding the current health care debate, I don't know if things are worse now than ever before, they might be. I don't know if the bill (or bills) winding their way through Congress are good or bad. Mary Ad originally wanted to call her second book *The Truth Will Set You Free*. It is my hope that in reading *TLG*, you will have some sense of how to evaluate this or any future political debate (health care or something else), and you will look for what is not said, and ask, as the cynical optimist, "Why?"

www.ingramcontent.com/pod-product-compliance
Lightning Source LLC
Chambersburg PA
CBHW031458270326
41930CB00006B/152